No Milk

D1453222

Daniel A. Twogood, B.A., D.C.

Victorville, California: WILHELMINA BOOKS

Printed in the United States of America

Published by
Wilhelmina Books
P.O. Box SVL 8354
Victorville, California 92392

ISBN Number 0-9631125-0-3

Library of Congress Card Catalog Number 91-067487

Contents

Preface

I asked a couple of reputable doctors to read my work, then lend their famous names and a nice comment, signed by them, to be used as the preface of this book.

Well, I'm writing my own preface. You see, they each read the book, and one of them said, "I think that you have to be a little more formal and maintain a slightly greater degree of professional dignity. I also think that some of your criticism should be toned down some in order to prevent avoidable alienation of potential supporters in the healing professions. You hit the nail on the head but I think it would be best if you are a little more gentle with your criticisms."

You should know something about me before you read this book-lest you become offended. My professional dignity is on display daily in my office. Even though I don't wear a white coat or a tie, I listen to my patients. I address their physical complaints and questions with patience and thoroughness. I make a concerted effort to determine the cause of their symptoms, then eliminate them so they don't need me anymore. I don't believe people need doctors, and because of that attitude, doctors might be offended if they read this book. They might also be offended because I criticize the medical professions.

But this book is not for doctors. It's for patients. It's for people who have already consulted doctors and found no answers. I published this book myself so I wouldn't be censored. I don't want to "tone down" my criticism, because I think it is accurate. If you're a patient, then you've been to doctors and you know. You know that medical services cost way too much—I mean **way** too much. They make you wait way too long for them to see you. For what they charge, you'd think they would be nice to you. You'd think they'd listen to you, concentrate on what you are saying. You might expect them to be polite to you. Sometimes they are, but not often enough. For all the money they charge, you would expect good results most every time.

Medical care is a necessity for many, but for many an unaffordable necessity. Meanwhile, doctors live lavish lifestyles. You'll see their Mercedes in the parking lot. They live in mansions while the masses who think they need them wait for hours and hours to be told they can't afford treatment. This is American medicine, and I'm sorry, but I am critical of it.

The fact is, results from medical treatment are not that good. Because of this, and doctors know it, you would think these same doctors would be open to new ideas. In my experience, they are not. So I'm critical of the medical profession. You think a doctor is going to put this book down because I criticize him, or what he or she stands for? No way. They won't even pick it up! So I'm not worried about what they might think. This is for patients who refuse to "live with their pain" like their doctors have advised them. And this book is for students who still have open minds.

Maybe my writing is a little rough. Well, I used to drive a forklift and supervise grocery warehouse workers, and I'm proud of that. I got to rub elbows with other working men, think their thoughts, live their lives, sweat their sweat, and talk their talk. So sometimes I say "ain't," and sometimes I see things and write about them in a different way than other published doctors.

But the message of this book is the truth. I'm about to tell you what I have seen in my practice. It's not what I was taught in school. It's not what you will read anywhere else. So, if you suffer from back pain, neck pain, and or headaches, read on. You are about to be rid of them.

Acknowledgements

I would like to thank my wife Willy, for her patience and guidance through this project. It was Willy who kept me from compromising my message.

Special thanks is due to my secretary Ana, who kept the salesmen away so I could work.

Thanks to Doug Dunn of Word Wizards who held my hand through the paper maze of publishing and printing.

The cover artwork is by Robbie Erwin. I think he did a great job.

And many, many thanks are due to all the patients who have consulted me, who listened to my ideas, and followed my instructions despite their doubts.

Dedication

This book is dedicated to the patients: those that have found no relief from their suffering, those who will find the answers in this book, and those who won't.

These are the patients who will teach me how to be a better doctor.

This book is especially dedicated to Robert Ester. He taught me to listen to patients. He taught me that patients often know more than doctors. Robert Ester changed my practice and changed my life.

Introduction

This book was not written because I'm a writer trying to get my first book published. I am not a writer. I am a chiropractor. I have been practicing for nine years, motivated by a sincere desire to help my patients live a life without pain in the best health possible. Being a health care practitioner is not easy. It's not like fixing toasters. The human body is much more complicated than a toaster. Not only that, but what the entire health care profession knows about the human body is very minimal when you consider what we don't know.

I'm not a genius. I'm not smarter or better than all the doctors in the country. I'm also neither a fanatic nor a salesman, although I feel like I am after five years of trying to convince people, doctors and patients, of my findings. Like I tell my patients, I did not make up what I am about to tell you. I studied very hard in school. I was actually an over-achiever. I learned everything I could — all the most minute, trivial facts about chiropractic, health care, and how the human body works. I did not put this knowledge together to come up with my findings . Instead, I have applied what I learned in school to this thing I kept seeing over and over again in practice, to try to explain it anatomically and physiologically.

You see, as any practitioner will tell you, theoretical medicine and clinical medicine, or health care, are two different things. Medical textbooks serve only as guidelines to the practicing physician. The practice of medicine has been an accumulation of experiences in the clinical setting based on the tried and true method we all use in real life — trial and error. We were all told things by our parents, things based on their experiences, that represented the truth and were given to us so we wouldn't make the same mistakes they made. But the joy of being a teenager is founded on making mistakes. Most of the time, we found that our parents were right, and after the cast was removed, or we were bailed out of jail, we felt we had verified what they had told us all along.

Most of the time, the accumulated medical experience related to the practitioner in textbooks, is true and repeatable. If a doctor sees a classic rash, a fever, or sees specific chemical changes in a blood sample that have been recorded by other practitioners over and over again, he doesn't have to be a maverick and get creative with a treatment program. Those who have gone before him or her have already done that. They have documented what works and what doesn't work. Believe me, many of them have already been creative beyond the call of duty, bless their souls. Doctors have tried bleeding diseased blood with leeches, frontal lobotomies for misfits, or applied beefsteaks to blackened eyes. They have tried injecting dyes into the spinal fluid to look for disc protrusions.

Many practitioners plug away in practice never deviating from conventional techniques. These are the good, safe doctors. If they do what the textbooks say, they will never have to worry about getting sued for malpractice, no matter what happens to the patient. Patients should understand malpractice law. According to law, it doesn't really matter what happens to the patient, as long as the doctor practiced good, safe, textbook procedure. If the patient dies, or is maimed, then it is not the doctor's fault, but a shortcoming of conventional medicine. These things happen, and sometimes even the best practitioner in the world will fail. There is no doctor in the world that gets 100% results. Most will get good, conventional results.

The problem with conventional medicine is that it gets conventional results. Statistics based on previous experience allows the practitioner to give you the going odds on your chance of recovery, or positive response to his treatment. Some procedures and treatment programs have excellent histories. This allows the doctor to give the patient a good prognosis, or prediction of outcome. Most doctors are very smart, but they cannot predict the future. They can only tell you what they have seen in previous cases like yours. Statistics and odds aren't really all that comforting to you, though, if it is your hide or life that is on the line.

"Gee, you just happen to be that one in a thousand that ended up paralyzed," does nothing to make that unlucky patient feel any better.

Conventional medicine has a pretty good track record for the simple stuff like broken bones, cuts, colds, etc. Or so it seems. In my opinion, most ailments will get better on their own without medical intervention. Many people feel obligated to visit the doctor when they get the sniffles, the flu, or a cough. In most of those cases, medical intervention will not change the course or outcome of the disease. However, most doctors feel obligated to intervene or manage these cases. After all, the patient is paying good money, so usually the doctor will give them their money's worth by filling out a prescription. However, most doctors realize that they have a plethora of cases in which the best treatment is no treatment at all, but they feel obliged to suggest some poisonous pharmaceutical to appease the patient.

You see, medication is seldom the true answer to returning a patient to health. The most glaring weakness with conventional medicine is that it deals only with end results, that is, naming the disease and prescribing a treatment program. Most disease processes are given a fancy Latin or Greek name that make doctors sound like they are smarter than the patients they are treating. Once that disease has been identified and named, the dictates of conventional medicine will spell out the preferred treatment, which, in most cases, is a chemical poison.

Conventional medicine almost always fails to address what seems to me to be the most obvious question: what is the cause of the disease?

In most cases the cause is obvious. A broken arm caused by falling off a horse is very easy to ascertain. It seems pretty self explanatory when flu symptoms begin when it is "going around." A patient with emphysema who smokes three packs a day needs only to read the pack of cigarettes to find the cause of his or her problem. Statistics have shown us that overweight, sedentary smokers have a tendency for heart disease. These things we know.

But some explanations just don't wash. When the flu is "going around," why do some people get it and some don't? Certainly in a household of six people, two of whom are sick with an airborne virus, all six have been exposed. But it is not always the case that all six get sick. What is the cause of the flu symptoms in the sick ones? What kept the well ones from getting sick?

What happened to Arthur Ashe, Pete Maravich, Jim Fixx, and Hank Gathers? These young world class athletes did not fit the typical heart patient profile, yet each of them had their well conditioned hearts fail for no apparent reason. Sure, autopsies and tests revealed occluded coronary arteries, but what caused those arteries to become occluded? They certainly weren't overweight, or sedentary. None of them smoked.

As a chiropractor, I treat patients with back pain, neck pain, and headaches. Let's be honest. The conventional results with conventional medicine for these disorders is extremely poor. Conventional treatment from the medical profession for these disorders is very limited. The usual medical procedure is very lopsided, with most of the time and expense concentrated in the area of diagnostic tests. Most doctors want to use their big microscopes to get some detailed pictures of the problem areas. You would have to sell your car to pay for the MRI's

(Magnetic Resonance Imaging) and CT (Computerized Tomography) scans and x-rays that most doctors will order. It seems such great expense would lead to a detailed treatment program, but if you've been through these procedures, you know that that is hardly the case.

Medical doctors can prescribe medication for pain and inflammation. In some cases these drugs will limit discomfort while the body heals itself. That describes the scenario of a successful case. Most of these medications cause more troublesome side effects than they alleviate. Medication is poison. The human body is a closed chemical system. Any time a foreign chemical is dumped into this system, the delicate chemical balance of the human body will be upset. This upset will manifest itself as side effects. All drugs cause side effects, no matter what your doctor tells you (or doesn't tell you).

I think everyone who is willing to take medication should own a *Physician's Desk Reference*. This book (called the PDR) comes out every year in a desperate attempt to keep up with the creations of the pharmaceutical companies. It lists all prescription medications on the market at the time. The PDR names these medications and lists their indications, contraindications, their chemical structures, and includes a color picture of each pill. The biggest section under each drug is called "Adverse Reactions." Do you think that doctors were aware of these adverse reactions before some poor patient experienced them?

Absolutely not. The practice of medicine has always been based on that old reliable tool that all of us use daily: trial and error. Trials that produced the desired results made it to the pharmacies. Many of those drugs were later pulled off the market when patients experienced adverse reactions that the poor lab animals didn't. When adverse reactions, or unexpected reactions produced some desirable symptom, a new drug was born. For example, one drug company recently developed a drug for heart patients that unexplainably produced hair growth in balding men. Now they are selling it like hotcakes for this side effect. So if you are bald, take this wonder drug. It may work. Of course, like most medications, no one knows why. You may get hair growth, but what in the world is it doing to a healthy heart?

I once had a patient who had a lot of faith in conventional medicine. She had open heart surgery three times. The third time the doctors opened her chest cavity, they installed a pace maker. She didn't need one yet, but they figured she would eventually, and this would save them a trip. She took lots of pills each day for her heart condition. She had seen the same doctor for years. For some reason, he decided to change one of her medications. The first time she took it, she went out afterwards and played golf. After about three holes, she broke out in hives and blew up like a balloon. She called her doctor. He had neglected to tell her the precautions for taking the new drug: don't expose yourself to sunlight when taking this medication. Better have your own PDR.

A medical doctor can also prescribe physical therapy for back pain and other musculoskeletal disorders. This sort of treatment usually involves a long term program of weeks or months of multiple treatments of physical modalities like heat, ice, exercise, ultrasound (a form of deep heat), or other electrical modalities that burn, tingle, or twitch the affected muscles. In my opinion, any patient who responds to physical therapy was going to get better anyway. Physical therapy is designed to speed up recovery, especially for athletes who must return to action. If physical therapy is going to be successful, the patient can do it him or herself at home without the trouble and expense of long term application of physical modalities. I have seen patients visit a physical therapist three times a week for months to simply lie on hot packs. This treatment does not require the presence of any kind of licensed professional. In my opinion, it is a complete waste of time and money. Such innocuous therapy can be performed at home. A patient traveling back and forth from home to the clinic probably causes more damage than the treatment can help.

The only other tool a medical doctor has for back pain is surgery. Back surgery has a very poor track record. The most successful cases get relief from severe back pain or resultant leg pain, but continue to have problems in the future. Many of these patients continue to deteriorate until they end up under the knife again. Again, these are the good cases.

Prior to back surgery, every honest surgeon will tell the patient that the odds of success are 50/50, that is, maybe you'll be better, maybe you won't. A more accurate prediction is 33/33/33. Maybe you'll be better, maybe you'll be the same, and maybe you'll be worse. Where else besides major league baseball is a professional paid big bucks for that kind of success rate?

The reason for the poor success in back surgery is poor screening of patients, usually because of a poor or absent investigation into the cause of the symptoms. I once saw a patient for neck and upper back pain. During the course of treatment, he asked me what I thought about a lump on the side of his jaw. I told him he needed to consult a medical doctor. He did, and it turned out to be cancer of the parotid gland (the salivary gland that is affected in mumps). He was treated with chemotherapy and recovered. Two years later he came to see me for low back and leg pain. I took two x-ray pictures of his low back, saw nothing abnormal, and referred him for a bone scan and medical examination to rule out any relationship to his previous carcinoma. Those tests were negative, so I began chiropractic treatment. After two treatments, and no response, he felt he needed further consultation. (This is a good case of the patient knowing more than the doctor. He felt something was wrong, and it is my opinion that no one knows the human body better than the owner). I referred him to a neurosurgeon who determined that he needed disc surgery to repair what he felt was a ruptured disc. When the surgeon opened up the back, he found a cancerous lymph node. The disc was fine. Although I was wrong in my treatment, and the surgeon was wrong, this was a very successful case. The cause of the pain was determined and eliminated. But back surgery typically has poor results because laminectomy fusions are performed when that surgery does not address the cause of the pain. That particular surgery is often performed because that's what is usually done, and seemingly for no other reason. Sometimes it works, sometimes it doesn't, and since the doctors don't know what else to do, they give it a try. Many of these cases end up under the knife because they are experiencing severe pain. Most doctors and patients assume that severe pain means a severe disease process, therefor deserving of severe, aggressive medical intervention.

However, severe pain seldom indicates a severe problem. Most severe problems (that are not induced by severe trauma) present as more low grade, insidious pain. When a patient presents with severe, excruciating pain, many doctors will panic by proceeding with aggressive, non pointed intervention. When a patient is screaming, the doctors tend to react, "rush her to surgery! STAT!"

That reminds me of a scene in the movie, *One Flew Over the Cuckoo's Nest,* a movie about patients in a mental hospital. One of the patients becomes hysterical for no apparent reason. The orderlies grab him, force him to the floor, and sedate him because, presumably, he's crazy. It turns out one of the other patients had dropped a burning match in the cuff of his pants and he was merely in pain.

The cases of severe pain that exist for no apparent reason are cases that require quick, thorough investigation as to the cause. If the cause is not apparent, then pain medication is needed to get the patient out of pain, and to allow the doctor to gather his or her wits and make a decision based on concrete findings. Because of the poor results of back surgery, I recommend it only for the patient who has tried conservative treatment, has had no response, and is ready to put a gun to his head.

The most impotent medical treatment for back pain is actually the one most commonly recommended by doctors: "There is nothing that can be done. Learn to live with your pain. Eventually, when you can't stand it anymore, you'll need surgery." After thousands of dollars spent for so called "expert" medical care, this answer is totally unacceptable. If a patient wants to live with pain, then he or she should give up at this point. Cut your losses and use drugs for pain. But as long as a patient chooses to live, he or she should seek help. Get another opinion. I think more opinions are better. All a doctor has to offer is his or her opinion. A doctor cannot "order" a patient to do anything. Consider a doctor's advice, then make your own decision. It's your body. If your doctor gives you an order, get a new doctor.

So what is conservative treatment? Chiropractic is conservative treatment. I don't want to seem biased against the medical profession, but chiropractic care gets better results than medical care in most cases of back pain, neck pain, and headaches. Chiropractic care is a form of physical therapy — a very powerful form of physical therapy. Manipulation is the distinctive tool of chiropractic. The theory of chiropractic is that many cases of back pain, neck pain, and headaches are caused by the misalignment, or lack of mobility, of the moveable vertebrae of the spine. In chiropractic theory, these misalignments (called subluxations) cause pressure on soft tissue structures of the spine (discs, ligaments, and nerves) causing structural changes that can cause back pain, often radiating into the head, arms, hands, or internal organs. Most chiropractors will tell patients that, in order to alleviate symptoms, a series of treatments is necessary to accomplish the realignment of the spine. The axiom of chiropractic, that founding principle that sets chiropractic apart from conventional medicine, is that the **cause** of pain is investigated, determined, and eliminated. Almost all chiropractors will tell you that the cause of symptoms is some sort of spinal or pelvic misalignment.

That's a pretty good theory, and chiropractic treatment gets pretty good results. But if we examine the results in the great majority of cases, we see that most patients respond with short term or long term treatment, but eventually have a recurrence of the same symptoms over and over again throughout their lives. Those who have undergone successful indoctrination by a smooth talking chiropractor believe that they will **always** need chiropractic care. They return faithfully to their chiropractors for their weekly or monthly maintenance treatments, or whenever their usual symptoms flair up again.

I practice in a rapidly growing community in Southern California, consequently I see lots of new patients who have just moved to the area. Many of these people are looking for a new chiropractor to give them the lifetime treatment that they have been told they will always need. Many of them carry a little card from their chiropractor that lists the bones that keep going out of place, and what direction they need to be manipulated to alleviate symptoms, or cause correction, or something. Most of these people have been through the medical gamut of treatment for their problems, and have found that chiropractic care has given them the best results.

But when I question these people about their symptoms, I find some interesting things. First, I ask them what caused their pain. Most of them will report that their symptoms began shortly after some physically traumatic incident, like a fall, or an auto accident. When asked what helps their condition, they tell me that they tried lots of medications that didn't help, then discovered chiropractic. Chiropractic adjustments, they report, help. In my next question, I ask them if, over the years they have had the problem, has their condition gotten better, worse, or stayed the same. Almost all of these patients respond that they have not improved, or have gradually gotten worse, but that chiropractic treatment has always helped. The usual justification from the chiropractic profession for these results, is that these patients would be much worse, maybe even in wheelchairs, if not for chiropractic care. Boy, that would make you keep up your visits to the chiropractor, wouldn't it?

I don't want to sound cynical about all health care professionals. Sometimes accidents or poor health habits cause irreversible changes that require perpetual treatment. Sometimes. If you smoked your whole life and end up with emphysema as a result, you will require oxygen and or respiratory therapy to keep you alive. If you played football and damaged cartilage in your knees, you may require repetitive surgery, physical therapy, or drugs for pain for years to come. But to require lifetime chiropractic or drug treatment because once you bent over and sneezed, or once your car was rear ended, or once you vacuumed the floor and your back "went out" defies logic. Isn't the human body more resilient than that?

I think so. For God's sake, some people fall out of buildings and recover. One man fell out of an airplane at 23,000 feet and hit the ground. Sure, he broke every bone in his body, but he lived, and eventually walked and talked and jumped out of airplanes again.

In my opinion, ongoing chiropractic care is no more useful than aspirin. Well, there are no side effects to manipulation, despite what medical doctors will tell you. So chiropractic care will, in many cases, help you to feel better for the time being. But chiropractors claim to address the **cause** of pain, and eliminate it. What happened to that? What happened to the elimination of the cause, and therefor further treatment? There are some chiropractors who try to get rid of patients by truly permanently eliminating the cause of symptoms and therefor treatment. But most chiropractors try to **keep** patients, by selling them on the need for regular care, or maintenance care, or at least a return to their form of treatment when the inevitable recurrence happens. These doctors have convinced patients that treatment is keeping them out of wheelchairs. There are whole seminars on how to keep patients coming. I don't want to imply that chiropractors are unethical, although **many** are. Lots of chiropractors actually believe what they tell their patients, in fact most of them believe it. But many chiropractors prescribe treatment programs based more on their own financial needs than on what their patients need. Maybe I'm a traitor, but I have talked with a lot of chiropractors, and this phenomenon is not a rare occurrence.

Although there are lots of bad apples in the chiropractic and medical professions, in fact in **all** professions, I honestly believe that most doctors act basically in good faith. We just don't know any better, and that's not a condemnation. We honestly just don't know any better. Like I said, what we health care professionals know about the human body is minimal when you consider what we **don't** know.

So, to get unconventional results, that is, to effect the **cure** of disease, we need to look to unconventional medicine. We need to consider those maniacs on the fringe of conventional medicine. And believe me, there are some maniacs out here. But I love them because they are seeking the truth, they're walking point, they're risking their credibility in the hope of improving on conventional results.

Check out Kevin Costner in the beginning of his epic film, *Dances with Wolves.* A stalemate battle situation moved him to insane actions that got good results. Conventional battlefield practices were getting nowhere, so he went out on the fringe. He risked failure, but succeeded. He tried something daring to create a change. He was shooting in the dark, but it worked.

Are we on the fringe of medicine shooting in the dark? Yes, but not totally. Usually we invade the dark because we saw a glimmer out there. Maybe a fleeting glimmer, but we **know** we saw something.

All through the beginning years of my practice I was bothered by the cases that I know all chiropractors have seen: those patients that are experiencing sudden acute pain, for no apparent reason. The key words here are "no apparent reason." These patients commonly would tell me that they had severe low back pain after merely bending over to pick up the newspaper.

Okay. That could happen. I was taught in school that severe low back pain is caused by bending, lifting, twisting, or falling. Many patients relate that they bent *wrong,* or slept *wrong,* or twisted *wrong.* Well, based on their condition, you would have to say that *something* was *wrong.* But when you pick up the newspaper every morning for years *right,* what in the heck did you do **this** time that was so *wrong?* It's not such a hard thing to do. It seems you would have learned such a simple task *right* by now. What gives?

I know, I know. I was taught that if I take a thorough history of the patient's activities over the weeks prior to the onset of pain, I will surely find a strenuous episode that could have caused the damage that eventually lead to this acute pain. When I discovered that the patient lifted a refrigerator two weeks before he or she felt pain, I feel the cause is now *apparent*. I then tell him or her my shoelace story. It's a really good story. It goes like this:

When you buy a new pair of tennis shoes that you wear every day, you begin each day by tying the laces. You pull on these laces in the same way, with the same force that you always have, literally thousands of times. You've done it so many times you could do it in your sleep. You never do it *wrong*. But after years or months, usually when you're in a hurry to go somewhere, and you're already late, and your friends are all waiting, and they're already mad at you, and you have a headache anyway, you tug on your laces like you always have, and they break.

Don't you hate that? I do.

Well, the guy who threw his back out bending over for the newspaper **really** did the damage when he lifted the refrigerator. I usually explain that the stress of that lifting tore some of the fibers in the outer part of one of his discs (the pads between the vertebrae). Bending over for the newspaper each day brought him closer and closer to that inevitable day when the disc exploded through those torn fibers.

It could happen.

But then there were the cases for which I had no shoelace story. These people experienced severe pain after having done **nothing.**

"Really?" I would ask.

"Nothing, absolutely nothing," they would say. "I went to bed last night feeling absolutely fine. When I woke up this morning, I couldn't get out of bed."

Further investigation into their activities over the last few weeks reveals nothing. Well, as a doctor, I don't have any qualms about saying I don't know what's going on. Any doctor should feel comfortable saying that. I once had a really good teacher in high school who used to say that a lot. All the kids liked her and had great faith in her, because she was like us, she didn't know sometimes. But I think we really looked up to her because she never said just "I don't know."

She always said, "I don't know, but I'll find out."

What a great teacher. She always did, too. She got back to us.

In these cases with no apparent cause, and there are lots of them, a thorough investigation didn't reveal a satisfactory answer to justify the pain. I always proceeded with these cases with chiropractic treatment, and they usually got better, but I was always bugged by them.

"No apparent cause." That phrase, and these cases kept bouncing around in my head.

Modern medicine has made many technological advances in the last 20 years. We have better diagnostic techniques. We have gone beyond x-ray to computerized tomography (CT scans) and magnetic resonance imaging (MRI) for more detailed, more accurate images of tissue. We can look very closely at tissue to determine what microscopic changes have occurred. Our blood testing has become more detailed and reliable. We have bigger and better microscopes. Everything is computerized. **Where** we choose to look, everything is more apparent. But despite our better, more technological diagnostic tools, the causes of some conditions are just not apparent.

What is it then? Why do so many diseases have causes that are unknown, or not apparent? We can describe the tissue changes of lupus erythematosis, but the cause of the disease is unknown. The same goes for multiple sclerosis. All we can really say for sure is, "Yep, we've seen that before." Medical textbooks are full of diseases that we can describe to a T, but for which we know of no cause and no treatment.

So many cases of back pain are the same. Patients present with severe pain, but x-rays and CT scans are negative. The images in these tests are perfectly clear, the tissue is highly detailed. Doctors couldn't ask for better quality information. But it is negative!

I don't care how big or expensive your telescope is, you will not be able to see the sun at night. Assemble all the best astronomers in the world to look for the sun at night and none of them will see it. The same is true for these "no apparent cause" cases of back pain, neck pain and headaches. Many patients assume that if they carry their x-rays and blood tests and CT scans around from doctor to doctor, they will eventually find that great doctor who will cure them with his superior skills in diagnosis. I've had patients tell me that they found a doctor who took "more extensive" x-rays.

Good for him. What happened? All the other great doctors didn't look close enough? Is he or his x-ray machine so much better that he's going to see something everyone else missed?

I want to make a statement here: X-ray is an over-rated diagnostic tool. When a patient goes to the doctor with back pain, you can bet x-rays will be taken. Everyone, doctors and patients, assume that the answer to their back problems are going to appear on that black and white film. That is a huge assumption.

The doctor carefully scans the film with his well trained eyes.

"Hmmmmmmmmmmmm." (Doctor talk).

If anything abnormal appears on that film, then that's it. That's the cause of the pain. That again is a huge assumption.

"Ah HAH! Arthritis!" or God knows what.

But, God forbid the x-ray appears negative (which it often does) ... no apparent cause.

When there is no apparent cause, and all the best doctors in the world are huddled around the x-rays, none of them are going to solve the case. It's going to be the guy in the next room who hollers out, "Hey you guys, come take a look at this!"

That's right folks, the doctor on the fringe is going to solve the case if anyone is. It's not going to be a better drug, or a better spinal manipulator, or a better pair of eyes. Sure, each expert will come up with a fancier diagnosis, but that won't solve the case. It's going to be the guy who took a different approach who solves the case.

It's going to be the guy in the back of the x-ray room that thought he saw a glimmer out of the corner of his eye. When he did a double take, the glimmer was gone, so he stared some more with the others at the x-rays. No matter how hard he looked at those films, he saw nothing. Then there was that glimmer again, he thought, but maybe not. Maybe his eyes were just tired.

No, there it is again.

"Hey you guys, did you see that over there?"

The others looked at him annoyed. "What in the world are you looking at? Any idiot knows you're not going to see anything over there. The view box is up here!"

Finally, he grew annoyed with the pointless staring at that x-ray film. He saw that glimmer again, and this time he followed it into the darkness of the next room. The fluorescent glow of the x-ray view box faded behind him as he slowly moved after that glimmer, deeper into the darkness of the next room. The incredulous comments of those other doctors faded behind him as he concentrated on the glimmer ahead of him now. It was so hard to see at first. He had to concentrate so hard just to keep it in view. Sometimes he wasn't even sure he was seeing anything real.

Soon he was in the next room, not far from the others. The glimmer was now a bright light sitting on the table before him just as clear as could be. He never even thought to look in this room for the answer, but there it was. Any one of those other guys could have seen it, but no one thought to come in here.

He rushed back to the other room. He could barely contain his excitement. He had seen the truth and he wanted to share it with the others.

"Hey you guys, I found it, the answer! It's in this room over here!"

The others couldn't believe him. They looked at each other in disbelief, then at him with disgust.

"We've been looking for the answer a lot longer than you have! We know the answer cannot possibly be in that room. The x-ray view box is over here!"

"Just come look!" he cried desperately. His excitement was turning to panic. He looked back over his shoulder into the other room to make sure the light was still there.

"We refuse to insult our intelligence by taking the trouble to walk over there" snipped the leader of those other doctors, as he stomped out his cigarette in disgust.

Finally he gave up on convincing the others. He went back into the other room and concentrated on the light. "Well", he thought to himself, "I guess I'll take this to the patient. I hope he doesn't refuse to look at it."

The answer to these cases is in the other room. It's not always easy to see, at least in the beginning, but you have to look in that direction. The approach of conventional medicine is to build bigger and better microscopes and keep looking in the same direction. This only leads to nearsightedness and closed mindedness. Yes, the doctor on the fringe is the one who is going to see the truth.

I was lead onto the fringe of medicine in 1985 by Robert Ester.

Thank God for Robert Ester.

1

The Cause of Disease

Did you know that most of the disease of men, and women, and children is caused by the foods people eat?

If you've ever heard that before, you are well read in either really new health literature, or really old health literature. In between old and new we got smart. So smart that we missed the point. So smart that our health got worse. So smart that the health care professions got completely off track.

Hippocrates, who was born in 460 B.C., compiled the first modern medical literature. Hippocrates believed that much healing came about from "the effort of nature." He wrote the Hippocratic Oath which is the solemn oath of medical practitioners today. In this oath, he swore that, as a health care practitioner, he would give no "deadly medicines." He said: "The key to health is through natural living."

For many years after Hippocrates established the Hippocratic oath, medical practitioners were satisfied to use natural remedies to restore health to the human body. Then, about the beginning of the 16th century, a German physician named Theopratus von Hohemheim went into the mines at Tyrol where he saw minerals being purified by other minerals. He began using minerals on his patients, assuming they could purify their bodies in the same way. After von Hohemheim, other practitioners began experimenting with minerals.

Louis Pasteur is the father of modern medicine. He invented microbiology and immunization. He believed in sterilization, inoculation, and surgery to correct the ills that begot man. He worked with an understudy, a protégé named Antoine Beschamp. Beschamp viewed the solution to disease in a more "preventative" rather than "patch them up" approach. He chose to attack disease from the cause end rather than from the effect end. He came up with his five tenants of health:

1) Get a moderate amount of rest.
2) Get a moderate amount of exercise.
3) Eat a nutritious, balanced diet.
4) Drink pure, clean water.
5) Breathe pure, clean air.

His opinion, and mine, is that if all of us practiced these five tenants from the womb to the grave, most of the exercises doctors go through to practice modern conventional medicine would be unnecessary.

Most people view physicians today as the knowledgeable leaders in the quest for optimum health. Most physicians began medical school with a sincere desire to become well educated so they could diagnose, advise, and lead their patients to optimum health. But by the time they have spent eight years being indoctrinated by the A.M.A. (American Medical Association) and the pharmaceutical companies, most physicians have become nothing more than glorified drug pushers. The American public's view of health care places the physician on a pedestal as a being who is all-knowing about what ails the human body. Once he or she has tested, probed, prodded, and examined you thoroughly, a diagnosis is reached. Then, this all-knowing physician has access to the huge apothecary in the sky (or the new, free samples in his desk drawer). Your optimum health returns to you after his or her judicious choice of drugs. The correct pill will fix you up.

No Milk

Although this terrible fallacy is slowly being dispelled by an increasingly aware and better educated public, this erroneous view of health care is still rampant in the general public. Nothing could be further from the truth. The truth is, perfect health becomes compromised, or less than perfect, by four different causes:

1) Inheritance of genetic weaknesses or abnormalities.
2) Trauma (falls, accidents, etc.)
3) Exposure (infection, ingestion, inhalation, inoculation, or contact)
4) Unknown causes.

There will always be unknown causes. I keep saying it, but, what we physicians know about disease and the human body is minimal compared to what we don't know. Many times, when you take your car to the mechanic, he has a difficult time determining what is wrong with it, and he is working on a system that was designed and built by man. Physicians don't have that luxury. Most of what we know about health care has come about by trial and error — a lot of error.

Most medical doctors who practice conventional medicine view the human body as a chemical playground. Since von Hohemheim, they have discovered that symptoms can be manipulated, or changed, by adding some chemical to the bloodstream. Sometimes, an undesirable symptom is eliminated. Usually, though, another **un**desirable side effect is created. When this happens, conventional medical wisdom dictates that **yet another** chemical is added to the bloodstream to counteract the side effect of the first chemical. This can go on for ever. I have seen these patients. They have a purse full of plastic bottles. Many times their main complaint, for which they are consulting me, is merely another side effect of the poisonous chemicals their doctors have prescribed.

So the foundation of modern medicine today is to diagnose disease through thorough testing, then **add** chemicals until the desired effect is attained. In my opinion, this form of treatment is moving in the exact opposite direction that it should be moving. The starting point should definitely be thorough testing. But most conventional doctors use testing to come up with a diagnosis, a fancy Latin or Greek name. Once the name is established, the textbooks and previous experience dictate treatment, usually drug therapy.

Also, most modern diagnostic testing involves batteries of blood tests, x-rays, and other high-tech techniques. This is the area in which modern medicine has made the most advances. We can use some really expensive equipment to get some really detailed information, but so what? The only change this affects is a higher medical bill. The diagnosis is the same, so the doctor proceeds with the same treatment. Granted, pharmaceutical companies are always developing new drugs, but again, this just moves the case in the same direction, that is, **adding** chemicals to change symptoms.

Modern medicine needs to move backward about 2000 years. In those days electronic, high-tech equipment was not available. Doctors didn't sit behind desks, read computer print outs, then write out a prescription. They looked at the patient, they talked to the patient, they asked lots of questions. Then they got up, they walked around that stupid desk and took a closer look. They actually touched the patient. They put their hands and their ears on the patient.

This is health care. The most powerful diagnostic tool requires no electricity. It requires only an attentive, caring ear. A well trained doctor who **listens** to the patient and asks well designed, pointed questions will stand a better chance of solving those tough cases, and not screwing up the simple ones. A thorough history is the most powerful diagnostic tool available to any physician. The goal of a thorough history, unlike high-tech tools, is not merely a diagnosis, a fancy name, but to determine the **cause** of the pain or disease.

As a chiropractor, most of the patients I see complain of neck pain, back pain, and/or headaches. I was taught in school that these conditions are almost always caused by trauma to the spine, like bending, lifting, twisting, falling, auto accidents, or wear and tear over time. The first order of business in handling these cases, like any other medical case, is a thorough history to determine when this traumatic event occurred and what damage it caused. Well, sometimes, as I said before, and as all chiropractors have noticed, sometimes there is no previous trauma to justify the patient's condition. This would lead one to believe that perhaps these conditions can be caused by something else. Well, we are taught a lot of these "something else's" in school. Other causes we are taught to consider are infectious diseases, tumors, or referred pain from other organs.

For example, low back pain can be the main complaint in a patient who is passing a kidney stone. Tubal pregnancies or ovarian cysts can cause low back pain. So can countless disorders. But after these are eliminated, there are still plenty of cases of back pain, neck pain, and headaches that have no apparent cause. We are obviously missing something.

Well, I have discovered that the main cause of back pain, neck pain, and headaches is of dietary origin.

"Say what?"

Okay. Let's get straight to the point. The most common cause of back pain, neck pain, and headaches is casein (one of the proteins found in cow's milk).

I didn't make that up. Honest. I couldn't have thought of that. I just happened to see it. I was told by Robert Ester to look for it, and, thank God, I did. I looked, and there it was!

I wouldn't have believed that seven years ago.

I don't make that statement without having made pretty darn sure that it's true. I wouldn't make such a statement, one that goes totally against everything I was taught ... that statement goes totally against the grain of conventional medical thought ... without checking it out.

You know, if you are totally out of stock of your best seller, but the computer says you have lots, you better check every possibility before you lay that kind of news on the guy who signs your check!

Well, my patients sign my checks. I put my heart out there for my patients. I want only one thing when I take on a case: to get that patient out of pain ... once and for all. Determine the cause, eliminate it! Period.

Now that I have discovered that the main cause of neck pain, back pain, and headaches is casein, I really have to stick my neck out. I almost always have to tell them this new notion ... my discovery.

You know what? I have had patients walk into my office, who have been to lots of doctors and chiropractors, and tell me that they want to come see me two or three times a week for adjustments, because adjustments help. Their checkbooks are open, their minds are made up. They want to make my car payment!

You see, they first consulted a physician, an M.D., you know, a real doctor. He ran lots of tests, then prescribed medication. Several years later they still suffer, plus they have an ulcer from the medication! So, out of desperation, and against their better judgement, they decide to appease their friends, and they quietly slip into a chiropractor's office.

"Come on, Sarah said it worked for her!"

So now, after moving all over the country and seeing lots of chiropractors, who have all agreed that this patient needs perpetual care, they have come to see me.

They carry a little business card with a chiropractor's name, and a list of their subluxations, that is, the bones that keep going "out of place". They want to come in to see me ... and pay me ... several times a week ... forever, to keep putting those bones back in place.

Wow! What a great profession! You mean, all I have to do is "crack" their bones once in a while, like, forever? And make lots of money?

You know, money is okay. We all need it. But it's just a vehicle, it's just a means of exchange. And if you get motivated by it, well, you lose your train of thought. So, I have an office manager, so I don't have to deal with money. It clouds my thinking. And, when I'm trying to convince people to consider this different notion of mine, so they can live without pain, well, that's all I can do.

So I discovered that casein is the main cause of back pain. That is, most cases of back pain are caused by a reaction to casein.

By the way, back pain as a major health problem, is unique to industrialized countries, like ours. The thought is that the onslaught of industrial type labor, totin' that barge, liftin' that bail, has caused back pain, the most common industrial injury. But the diets of industrial nations are also unique, especially with refrigeration and mass production. The heavy use of meat and dairy products is unique to industrial countries, like the USA. This great country is the richest in the world. We are the freest. We have the best health care in the world ... Right?

Well, I guess so. That's what they tell us. But let's observe.

All I do is observe.

Because I see lots of people who experience neck pain, back pain, and headaches, that is my specialty. So, I try to observe causal relationships. That is, what changed between the time that a patient felt okay, then, all of a sudden, experienced pain.

Well, like I said, we are the richest country in the world. We are the most technologically advanced country in the world. Right?

We got big microscopes.

We got nuclear medicine.

We got research.

We got the A.M.A.

OBSERVATION: How come, despite all of our great medicine, cancer has been on the increase since the turn of the century? How come heart disease, that was **not** a major problem in the 1800's, is now the **number one** health problem in our great country?

HOW COME?

Well, I think we're missing something. Yeah, we know we all need to lose weight, exercise, eat right, etc. All of us doctors practice this nice, safe, conventional medicine. Don't rock the boat, just adjust spines, prescribe medication, and go to the country club for drinks!

I would love to go to the country club.

But, I discovered that casein is the main cause of neck pain, back pain, and headaches! So I have to stay in my office and convince people to change their diets by eliminating foods that they love! I would love to tell them to avoid eating lima beans, liver, and spinach. But darn it, I have to peddle this discovery!

I have to!

I must!

Why?

Because it is the truth. That is ... casein is the main cause of neck pain, back pain, and headaches.

This determination I have made from experience, observation, study of relevant published works, and subsequent deduction.

I didn't make it up. I just happened to see it, after it was pointed out to me by a patient, a Mr. Robert Ester. He told me that his pain was due to certain foods in his diet. He told me that each and every time he ate dairy foods, he experienced headaches and back pain.

These thoughts are new, at least to me, and the future holds many changes in the theories I have deduced from the evidence. In the beginning, that was 1985, I searched diligently, without help, through the literature to see if someone else had seen what I was seeing. I used to frequent malls, and spend hours in book stores, reading the newest material in health care: books about arthritis, allergies, back pain, diet, etc. I found nothing. Nothing new, that is, or even suggesting that they were on to Robert Ester.

However, I continued to pursue this new area of study because, despite the fact that I found nothing in the literature to corroborate my findings, I was accumulating data in my clinical experience that left no doubt in my mind that I was on to something that was never a part of my formal education.

You see, I was taught that headaches, neck pain, and back pain are caused by trauma to the spine. This trauma causes structural, and subsequent physiological changes that produce symptoms. These symptoms, or changes, cause such discomfort to the victim, or patient, that they seek professional help. These changes can produce far reaching symptoms due to the pressure, electrical changes, or other physical changes to the spinal column that can affect the nerves that pass in, around, between, and through these bony structures. Most chiropractic techniques utilize some sort of manipulation of these bony structures that is designed to **reverse these traumatic changes** so that the symptoms are eliminated, or reduced.

Chiropractic philosophy dictates **that the cause of these symptoms is determined ... then eliminated.** That's a noble cause!!

So, the cause is assumed to be: subluxation, or, bone, or vertebrae out of the place it should be. It is manipulated back to where it should be, and symptoms are eliminated or reduced. When the vertebrae of the spinal column are in their proper places, symptoms are eliminated. **THAT,** is chiropractic theory.

It's a good theory. It works. Many chiropractors use different techniques of patient management, and many of them have different ideas about what actually happens as a result of spinal manipulation. But, chiropractic results are better than medical results.

Medics, (M.D.s) are taught to eliminate or reduce these symptoms through controlled chemical or structural changes, that is, medication or surgery. If the symptoms are caused by inflammation of a joint, muscle, or nerve, the treatment of choice is an anti-inflammatory drug, such as naprosyn, motrin, or tolectin. If muscle **spasm** is involved, a muscle **relaxant** is prescribed. You see, pharmaceutical companies are working day and night to develop chemicals that can effectively reverse, or shut down, unpleasant symptoms. If the structural changes are severe enough, or irreversible, the doctor will prescribe surgery to correct the problem.

People consult doctors because they are experiencing symptoms that are getting in the way of their lifestyles. Most people, like myself, who experience **no symptoms**, do not consult doctors.

"If it ain't broke, don't fix it."

Chiropractors however, that is, many of them, believe they can **prevent** symptoms with manipulation of the spine. The theory is that the subluxation precedes the symptoms. So by correcting the subluxations in a healthy person who is unknowingly about to become sick, disease can be prevented.

Prevention is the name of the game. We are all beginning to realize that, if we don't create a problem, we don't have to deal with it. This is true.

When you consult a physician because you can no longer breathe without concerted effort, what is it you want?

Relief, right? You want to be able to breathe.

But, if you have been smoking three packs of cigarettes a day, and you don't live in a cave, what is it you really want?

"Please doc, tell me it's not what I think it is, that is, what I've been reading about on all of those packs I smoke every day! I've already memorized that: 'The Surgeon General has determined that blah blah blah...' "

So, many people want to believe that they are not responsible for their own health. "Fix me, Doc. Please."

Let me tell you what I think about doctoring.

It is a tough profession.

Sure, doctors live in mansions on the hill, and drive exotic cars ... lots of them. Their wives, or ex-wives, flaunt excessive cars, jewelry, etc, all over town. They somehow manage to let you know that they have money.

But let me tell you what I think doctoring is all about:

Doctoring is a **partnership** between doctor and patient. Partnerships are tough. Each partner has a responsibility, at least one.

"You do your part, I'll do mine."

So, **I**, as a doctor, will give my best advice...

You, as a patient, must, **or should,** follow my advice. That doesn't mean I'm right.

You, as a patient, are paying for my opinion. I'm obligated to give you my opinion, no matter what I think you might think of it. My opinion may be wrong. If it's your judgement that my opinion is wrong, then that's your right. If a doctor suggests surgery, or drugs, or a diet change, it is your obligation as a patient to consider the opinion, then make your decision, whatever it is.

I want people to leave my office and follow my recommendations, **or consider me WRONG.**

You know, a lot of patients consider my advice **crazy.**

Well, that's a bummer!

I may be wrong, **but I'm not crazy.**

Just because my opinion is one you've never heard before, doesn't mean it's not true.

If medical knowledge is forever confined to our current knowledge, we are in big trouble. What do you think research is all about? The word is **RE**search. The first search didn't give us good enough results, so we've gotta search some more.

Until disease is totally stamped out, we better continue to consider ideas we haven't heard before. Because our current knowledge in the area of cancer isn't slowing it down. The same goes for heart disease and viral infections, like AIDS.

You know why?

Because, lots of patients have consulted lots of doctors, heard lots of diagnoses and stories, undergone lots of treatment, etc., and have had **NO** results. They have heard lots of diagnoses and undergone extensive treatment programs.

Many of these patients **want to hear the same story but get different results!**

What do they think when they come to consult me? That I'm such a better practitioner that I'll get better results using the same techniques?

No way.

I try really hard, but I'm no technician.

I just pay attention to results, and practice what gets that ... that is, results.

Manipulation of the spine is a powerful tool in health care. Before I began practicing bio-ecology (the study of how the human organism responds to environmental factors, like diet), I was a straight chiropractor and I got good results with manipulation of the spine. But, all of my patients didn't respond to treatment.

So, I obviously didn't know everything. And I still don't. Patients who didn't respond were referred to medics. Treatment then involved either drugs or surgery. The logic is that chiropractic is conservative care, and if a patient doesn't respond, more aggressive intervention is needed. You know, a bigger hammer. If that doesn't work, and it usually doesn't, what then?

End of medical and chiropractic knowledge? If the post surgical patient still experiences symptoms ... uh oh. What are the logical choices? Perform the surgery again?

Ask patients who have had multiple surgeries. An honest surgeon will tell you that your odds of improving after surgery are 50/50. With those odds, and one failure under your belt, do you really want another surgery?

No way.

The pharmaceutical companies will always have more samples. This, my friends, is not the answer either.

After chiropractic care has failed, and the orthopedists and neurologists are stumped, the usual procedure is to perform more tests. These tests are designed to find the needle in the haystack. But what if the needle isn't in the haystack? If the needle is in the pig's trough, the answer will not be found.

At this point, the case is progressing in the wrong direction. There are no more answers in additional tests, usually not even any good guesses. All the doctors are on their hands and knees in the haystack while some pig is screaming his head off with a needle in his bacon! But no one hears. The doctors will then get up, brush off their pants, and tell some one to shoot the pig. Then they'll look at you over their twisted bifocals and advise you to live with your pain, or consult a psychiatrist. If you are satisfied with "live with your pain", **then do it.**

I think patients should consider bio-ecology before they get cut and/or drugged. But, a patient who has run the medical and chiropractic gamut with no change in symptoms is my favorite patient. They have had all the bloody tests, and they are all negative. Good, that saves me some time. They want something different. I ask them, "do you want to hear the same story, then pray that I'm so much better that results will come about because I'm so skilled??"

I have met many medical and chiropractic practitioners. Almost all of them are sincere and want to help their patients. Almost all of them are proficient at what they do. Honest!

Every medical and chiropractic school has bad students that become bad doctors. But, that is not the problem. We need new ideas, new treatment programs, especially for those patients who cannot seem to get relief from their symptoms using conventional treatments.

What do you suppose the world record for the high-jump would be if athletes had insisted on the western roll technique? Dick Fosbury came along with his flop and revolutionized the event and the record. How many jumpers laughed at him then? Nobody's laughing now.

I began considering the bio-ecology approach in 1985 when it was handed to me on a silver platter by a patient.

Robert Ester, a 53 year old man, came into my office with shoulder pain that began after he worked on his car. In the course of my conversation with him (history), I asked him if he had ever experienced spinal problems.

He said, "Yes, I used to suffer from severe neck pain, back pain, and headaches for 30 years. I would experience episodes of burning pains that ran up and down my entire spine. I would have headaches so bad I had to stay in bed all day."

I said, "Did you say 'used to?' You don't anymore?"

"Nope, I'm cured."

I was taught in chiropractic school that the doctor does not "cure" disease. God, or Innate Intelligence, or Nature, or the Life Force, cures disease. It is the doctor's job to determine the cause of disease, then work with the patient to eliminate the cause. Then, the miraculous life force of the human body would "cure" the disease. That claim belongs to no mortal.

This, I firmly believe to this day. Dr. Dorothea Towne, D.C. taught me that, bless her soul. Bless her soul, and thanks to her for setting me off in the right direction. I'll never forget her. This is the foundation of chiropractic, and the foundation of my practice. It keeps me humble and at the business at hand.

So I react, usually in a negative way, when I hear that word, "cure".

"I'm cured."

Maybe my reaction is testimony to the poor results I had been getting in my practice. Sure, patients got better, but they were never "cured". They were lifetime patients. Those who suffered with chronic problems would always be back. I just helped them through a tough time, released them, then would see them several months or years later when the inevitable recurrence took place.

So Robert Ester had irritated me with his "I'm cured."

"So, what cured you?"

After I said it, I had hoped he hadn't noticed my tongue in my cheek. After all, I was just taking a history. I shouldn't be judging the man.

I was about to learn more about healing in this one conversation than I had learned in my entire formal education. I wish I had known it at the time.

First, talking to Robert Ester taught me to always have an open mind.

A closed mind learns only the hardest lessons.

What I was about to hear from Robert Ester, I was not going to believe. Thank God I was later to remember what he had said and, in a moment of desperation, give it some consideration. When I later discovered that he had spoken the truth, I decided to apply an axiom to my way of thinking:

Never dispute something that you cannot disprove.

"Well," he continued, (he didn't notice my doubts), "I saw chiropractors, orthopedists, neurologists, shrinks, everybody. They all performed lots of expensive tests and x-rays. Each one gathered the results and told me what he/she thought was wrong. Each one had some idea, and prescribed a treatment program. I got manipulated, I got physical therapy, drugs, analysis, the works. My symptoms never changed.

"But, along the way," he continued, "two doctors told me that tests had indicated that my cholesterol was slightly elevated. Although they each informed me that it had nothing to do with my back pain and headaches, I decided I would at least work on that. So, I changed my diet."

Pause.

I almost fell on top of him in anticipation.

"And?" I impatiently prompted, waving my hand in front of my open mouth.

You know, new doctors have the best chance of making the most of a patient's discovery. They have more time. At least, I did. I used to take naps between patients. If I had been busy, I would have proceeded with his treatment and dismissed his thoughts.

Maybe then, but not now.

You know what really gets my attention? When a patient says, "you know, doc, this may seem really weird, but..."

Now, when I hear that, I really listen.

You know why?

Because this patient thinks it is really weird, what she's about to tell me. But, whatever it is, it's real, because it keeps happening. It's not one of those things that happens once, or maybe it doesn't, you know, and you go, "Naw!"

They've checked this "thing" out, and they've seen it enough to realize it's not their imagination. They want to bounce it off someone, like a professional, and get some support for their sanity. The fact that they're mentioning it to you is significant:

"Tell me I'm not crazy, doc."

Robert Ester thought his case was weird, but he **knew** that what he had seen was the truth. He had checked it out. Thoroughly. He thought it was weird because he had been through all the tests. What he had discovered was never discussed. Surely one of the doctors would have figured out what he had figured out on his own.

"After I changed my diet, my pain went away."

Another pause while I looked to the upper corner of the room for the point I was obviously missing.

"So, you think something in your diet caused your pain?"

"Oh, I know it did."

"What was it?"

"Milk."

"Milk?"

"Milk. Well, not only milk, but everything that is made from milk, like cheese, ice cream, yogurt, all dairy products."

"What makes you think it was milk?"

No Milk

"Well, in order to lower my cholesterol I eliminated red meat, eggs, fat, all dairy products, sweets, and, well, you know, I really cleaned up my diet. After a few weeks, my pain went away. At first I didn't even notice. Then, I said, 'hey, I don't have a headache!' As the weeks went by I began to wonder 'what had changed?'

"Then, one day, after four months without pain, I got the urge for a glass of milk. I poured myself a big glass and began to drink.

"As the milk touched my lips, I experienced instantaneously a burning sensation up and down my spine. Within a few seconds I got a severe headache."

"I've never heard of that," I responded.

"Well, neither had I at that time. But that was several years ago. And since then, I have accidently, or in a moment of weakness, exposed myself to milk, or cheese, or cottage cheese, or some dairy product about 25 times. And each and every time it's the same ... back pain and a headache."

"Hmmmph." (Doctor talk)

"Once, my wife and I were out for a Sunday drive. We stopped at a donut store to get a donut. When I chose one, I asked the chef if it was made with milk. He assured me that it wasn't.

"We took our donuts home to have with coffee. When I took the first bite of the donut I instantly got back pain. I wrapped up the rest of the donut and, the next day, drove back to the donut shop. A different chef was working. I showed him the donut I had purchased the day before and asked him if it contained any milk. I told him that I had asked the Sunday chef the same question and he had informed me it did not. The new chef now before me apologized and said that the supplier had just changed the batter mix, and the new mix contained milk.

"That", he said, "is how sensitive I am to milk. One bite, and Wham!"

I thought this was an interesting story, but I really doubted that it was true. Something else must have changed to cause his symptoms to abate. Something that I knew about and understood. I'm a doctor, you know.

Maybe he was a head case.

The fact that I doubted his story has led me to understand and identify with my new patients when they give me that incredulous look after I tell them the "Robert Ester Story."

"Food can cause back pain? Give me a break!"

I wish, honestly, that what I had learned in school was true. I could go to work each day, do my (their) thing, then go home and relax.

But I can't. Sorry.

I have to be this weird guy and tell this weird story. It's like the movie, *Oh God*. In the movie, John Denver has this burden to bear. God has approached him and instructed him to spread the word that God is a little old man in a baseball cap. He knows it's true, because he has seen God, but he also knows that people think he's weird when he speaks the truth. Sigh. What to do. How do you convince people that the obvious is not true, and that something simple, but not obvious, is the actual truth?

Well, as far as I can tell, you stick with your feelings. You stick with what you have seen.

Voltaire said, "It is dangerous to be right in matters on which the established authorities are wrong."

People seem to want to cling to conventional thought. They have heard it so long, they **JUST KNOW** it's true.

You know, "feed a cold, starve a fever , put a beefsteak on a black eye, etc." People have been told in this country for decades that milk is good, healthy food. The dairy farmers have been very successful at promoting their products. They have lead us to believe that dairy products are not only healthy, but **ESSENTIAL** for our health. Without them, we would wither up and die. We would fall down and break if we didn't drink milk ... especially you women!

No Milk

Now some of us who read health magazines, know that, well, as adults, we can do without milk. But our kids **must have milk!**

Shouldn't they?

No.

How can I say this delicately?...I guess I could, if I had some manners, and didn't want to offend anyone. But, I seem to offend people anyway. Especially people who think, **or know,** that milk "Does a body good."

Who told them that?

Certainly **not** someone who might make some money from the sales of milk products!!?

Yeah, that's who. The dairy farmers.

Okay. Let's get this over with ... **Cow's Milk is not good food. Milk is terrible food. Milk does not do a body good. Milk causes, all by itself, more damage than any other supposed health food on the market. Milk is not good for kids, or adults. Cow's milk is designed for, and only good for ... baby cows! Milk is the number one cause of back pain and headaches.**

You can quote Dr. Twogood for that information.

Sorry. I wish I could convince you to read further without saying that. Lots of people salivate at this point. This certainly goes against what they have read, what all those old, smart, **experienced** doctors, **much more experienced doctors,** believe.

Who the heck am I?

Well, I'm this guy who saw something that is true, but goes against conventional medical thought.

I'm this guy who ran into Robert Ester.

You see, I didn't believe it either, when I heard it from Robert Ester. Why would he know something I didn't know? I'm a doctor, for God's sake! I studied this stuff!!

He's just a patient!

Just a patient!

Now, there's a mouthful!

No person knows more about the human body than the owner!

The patient!

That reminds me of a story I heard in Chiropractic School: The resident doctor was making his rounds in the hospital. He walked into the room of an 86 year old woman with a great smile. Anita.

The young doctor was tired. "God, another Alzheimer's case! I hope Karen wants Chinese tonight," he thought to himself.

He adjusted his stethoscope and placed the ice cold bell on the left side of her breastbone.

"I hope there's not any traffic in China Town!", he thought to himself.

He began to concentrate, then he felt her icy fingers tapping on his arm.

He looked up, perturbed, into her toothless grin.

"Excuse me young man, but my heart is on the right," she said, as she placed her left hand over her right breast, looking very patriotic.

The young doctor peered over his bifocals, thinking about Dim Sum and hoping he could order Chinese without appearing "uncool" to Karen. Thank God the entrees were numbered on the menu. He liked number seven.

He let go a cool smile.

"Sure. My heart's on the right too, and I don't know what the hell I'm doing!" he thought to himself, then glanced at his watch.

"Jesus!"

He continued, undaunted by her senile smile, closing his eyes to concentrate on her faint heart beat.

"Excuse me," she interrupted again. "But my heart is on the right."

She insisted on smiling that toothless grin.

The young doctor was obviously (but not to her, shoot, she was senile!) bugged.

She just kept smiling.

Well, the young doctor persisted, and she just kept tapping him with those cold, senile fingers.

He was somehow able to ignore her and get the hell out of her room.

"JESUS!"

He finally made it to the nurse's station to chart his work.

"God, I'm starving!" he thought.

He dropped the metal chart for Anita Quintanilla several times before he was able to pick it up for his last duty of the night.

"God," he swore.

When he flipped open the metal cover of Anita's chart, he knocked over a nurse's cup of coffee.

"Sorry," he said, realizing he was about done for the night, and ready to become the 'nice guy' for Karen.

He really felt compassionate.

His tired eyes scanned Anita's chart for the end of the doctors' scribbling that described her demise.

"Let's see." His eyes were about to fail him when they focused on those big red, underlined letters, scribbled by some other doctor before him who had been assigned to humor Anita.

"SITUS INVERSUS"

He dropped the chart and stared at the fluorescent light above the nurse's station.

He didn't want Chinese anymore.

He just wanted to be a good doctor, and he felt bad.

You see, situs inversus is a rare condition in which the internal organs of the human body are reversed. That is, the liver, which is usually on the right, is on the left. The stomach, usually on the left, is on the right, and the heart, usually on the left, is on the right! Just like Anita had told him. The internal organs are a mirror image of what is normal.

That's okay.

That look, that he thought was senile, it really wasn't. It was just the loving look of a sweet little old lady who was trying to be helpful. She probably looked at the young doctor with the same love and care she felt 60 years ago when she spoke to her then young son, who probably doubted her sincerity as much as the young doctor.

Makes you feel for Moms, huh? They do have a burden.

Well, can you imagine how this experience affected the young doctor?

I hope it affected him as much as Mr. Ester had affected me.

If it did, I would refer patients to him.

Wow.

Just when you think you know it all, you get zapped.

Thank God I got zapped.

I learned that some patients knew more than I did.

Boy, did that humble me?

I better not act so smart, because **I'M NOT!!!**

So, from that point on, I began, **CAUTIOUSLY,** considering that I just **MIGHT** be missing something! Maybe Robert Ester knew more than I did.

Now, after nearly six years of practicing bio-ecology (against the will of my patients) I feel like a Neanderthal. It seems the more I learn, the less I know. It's like putting together a jig saw puzzle of a clear blue sky.

I want all my patients to get better. I want them to realize why they have pain, then be able to eliminate the cause. But you know, there are lots of weaknesses with practicing bio-ecology.

No Milk

The first, and most obvious weakness, is my lack of understanding of this phenomenon. It has been right in front of our faces for decades, and only now are we, or at least some of us, taking a serious look at the relationship between diet and disease. Actually, doctors have noticed and studied the relationship between food and disease for nearly 50 years.

At first, I didn't believe Robert Ester. When I searched the literature I found nothing. But about four months after Robert Ester had told me about his case, I used what he had told me in a moment of desperation. I was seeing a patient who was failing to respond to treatment. Her symptoms seemed to come and go for no apparent reason. In a moment of frustration, I asked her if she drank milk. When she informed me she loved milk and drank lots of it, I told her the story of Mr. Ester. We decided to eliminate milk and dairy products from her diet and see what happened. Her symptoms disappeared in about one week. After two weeks of no pain, I instructed her to begin using milk again. Her pain returned four hours after her first glass of milk.

After this experience, I assumed that I had witnessed a rare allergy that would be useful in difficult cases. But after looking for the reaction for several years, I began to realize that the milk reaction was not rare, but very common. When I first noticed that Robert Ester was right, I thought to myself: "I better write a book before someone else sees what I see!"

I began writing this book in 1988. But at the same time, I have some friends who are professional health care practitioners. So I thought I should at least tell them, so they could help their patients. Honestly, that was my only motivation in telling them of my discoveries. I thought they would appreciate the info, and, at the same time, not steal my discovery and take credit for it.

Silly me.

Fortunately, my best friends remained that way, and just thought that I was experiencing a wild hair: "Dan's all right, just has a wild hair! He's done it before, but we still love him."

That was the best response. From my friends.

Others, even really good friends, thought I had crashed the barrier, you know, finally paid the price for being creative and different.

Now I throw my ideas out there as a joke sort of, you know, "here's the truth! Want some?"

Not many people do. Especially doctors. They want to hear something that fits comfortably into their beliefs. This notion somehow doesn't, so it is easily discounted.

So, the bottom line is, no one wants to steal the notion that back pain, neck pain, and headaches can, **and usually are**, caused by foods. They usually don't even want to accept it. They don't even want to **consider** it. Most of them don't even want to **hear** it!

So I grow another notch, I hope. So this book is for patients, not doctors. Doctors seem to know too much to consider this approach.

I really don't care that much that other health care professionals don't want to consider what I have seen.

I should, though.

It's kind of like Amway™, you know, network marketing. If I could convince a professional, who has access to lots of patients, the notion, or exposure, could grow in an exponential way. But, with professionals, egos get in the way.

I can understand that. When a patient considers another doctor's opinion more than mine, I salivate. I'm a product of the system too. I want to be right. I want to solve the case. Give me the credit. It feels good.

If a case doesn't respond like it should, that is, the patient doesn't get better, then, my responsibility is to refer the patient to another professional. I don't usually feel bad about that. I don't know everything, for God's sake! I need help once in a while!

But, I must tell you about this thing I have seen in my practice. I really don't believe that my discoveries will solve every case of back pain. Honest.

But, if a patient is going to pay for my opinion, then, by God, he, or she, ought to abide by the rules of our attempt. Many patients who don't respond to chiropractic manipulation, and dietary manipulation, later admit that they did not comply 100% with my suggestions.

Well, I don't want to be, or seem unreasonable, but if a patient doesn't follow my suggestions, and doesn't respond to treatment, well, I just have to assume only one thing, at least until proven wrong! Gosh darn, try what I have suggested. If it doesn't work, then we'll start over. This isn't a cure-all, it's a starting place.

But don't listen to what I have to say, then discount it, then wonder why you didn't respond to treatment!

I have had cases that didn't respond to treatment. I have had cases that did not respond to treatment and dietary manipulation. I have had cases that, I honestly felt, tried my suggestions and did not respond.

I relish those cases. If the patient can hang around long enough, get involved in the case, and follow instructions, we'll solve the case. We can learn more about disease and what causes it. That's how I got started onto the fringe of conventional medicine.

I was taught that back pain is caused by trauma. Then, I discovered that back pain can also be caused by reactions to certain foods in the diet, mainly milk and dairy products. Let's correct the physical changes caused by trauma with spinal manipulation. Let's correct the chemical changes with dietary manipulation. If that doesn't work, let's move into a new frontier with exhaustive investigation!

Who knows what else lies beyond our current knowledge?

Many times, I treat a patient with spinal manipulation and dietary manipulation and they respond! Wow! All right! I investigate the relationships between their symptoms and their diets and activities, then prescribe some changes. They get better. They're so amazed, they set up an appointment for their spouses. The spouse comes in with the same, or similar symptoms, and a similar diet.

"Gosh, I hate to sound like a broken record, but, you know what I told your wife? Well, I'm going to have to suggest the same changes for you."

Let's start at the top. This isn't magic. I ain't so smart, you know. I have to assume that what I've seen in my practice is true. That is, until we try what has worked before, in similar cases, we have to pursue this proven approach. If you follow my suggestions, (as generic and repetitive as they may sound) and you don't respond, then we'll try something else.

But many people want to skip to another approach, without trying the proven (at least to me) one. "Well, I want to get better, but I don't want to change my diet. That just sounds too far fetched!"

I once saw a patient who had gone through several back surgeries, had tried numerous medications, had seen every kind of doctor imaginable without any response. Her husband had seen me for chronic low back pain that completely disappeared when he quit dairy foods. She was a heavy milk drinker, but refused to give it up because it sounded too far fetched to her. Go and figure.

This is not a cure-all. This is not a far fetched notion. It's all about the observations I have made in my practice. I just look, pay attention, take notes, and tell you what I have seen.

You don't have to believe me. Just step away from the x-ray view box. Come into this other room. Look over here.

Now, you tell me ... What do you see?

2

The Milk Connection

In my practice, I have seen cases over and over again that have been through the medical gamut of treatments and have failed to respond. I have seen other cases that see doctors regularly for the same recurring symptoms. I have seen many of these cases respond merely by eliminating certain foods from their diets, mainly milk and dairy products. At first, I was baffled and amazed by what I was seeing.

First, I was amazed that musculoskeletal problems, that I had been taught to treat with physical medicine, responded to dietary changes. Secondly, I was amazed at how many different kinds of physical symptoms responded to these dietary changes. Third, I was most amazed at the fact that other doctors were not aware of this. I have seen patients who have been to the best doctors and clinics in the country with no results. I have seen patients who have had every test known to modern medicine with no results that would give them or their doctors the slightest clue as to what was causing their symptoms. I have seen patients who have had the most bizarre surgeries with no results. Mostly, I see patients who have a lifetime prescription for pain medication, and no hope.

What I have mainly seen, however, that prompted this book, is some classic symptoms that recur so frequently that they should be listed in medical books as pathognomonic for allergic reactions to foods, mainly dairy products. I have seen these symptoms in thousands of patients in the last six years. The following paragraph is a statement of fact. Six years after Robert Ester, this is where I have landed. Now, realize that the next paragraph is not taken out of, or derived from any textbooks. I did not make up what I am about to say. Like I said before, I am just an observer. The following statement is a description of what I have seen:

Most of the patients who come to see me complain of back pain, neck pain, and/or headaches. Almost all of these patients ingest dairy products as a regular part of their diets. In more than 90% of these cases, when dairy products are eliminated from the diet, back pain and headaches stop. When these patients begin ingesting dairy products again, their symptoms return.

Now, what does that mean to you? Well, if you had seen this phenomenon enough times, it would probably mean the same thing to you that it does to me. To me, it means this: the number one cause of back pain and headaches is milk and dairy products. But most people, upon hearing or reading that statement, think that it simply cannot be true.

Why?

Probably because they have never heard it before. No one ever told them that it **wasn't** true, but the logic of that statement seems to escape most people. Patients who have consulted lots of doctors have never heard it. Americans have been hearing for years that milk is good for them. They've been told that milk is essential for good health. In fact, they've been told that milk is good for bones, and since it seems their bones hurt, they **need** milk, or they may get worse.

They figure (I guess), how could such a young doctor know something that other older, more experienced doctors don't know? In fact, why would I know, or believe something that older more experienced doctors deny is true?

Well, because I lucked out, that's why. Robert Ester knew it, and he came in and told me about it, and I was just desperate enough to look at what he had told me. And when I looked, I saw it. It's really more complex than that, though. After observing the phenomenon for six years with lots of double takes and triple takes and eye rubbing and questioning and doubts, I've decided it's not a fluke, or even a rare occurrence. If you discover something new, you tell your best friends first.

"Hey, psssst, Dr. Goodfriend, who I went to school with for so many years. Guess what? Milk causes back pain. Yeah, no kidding. I'm not ready to tell anyone else yet, I'm writing a book, you know, but in the mean time, I'll let you in on the secret."

Don't you hate it when your friends roll their eyes at you with that "Yeah, right" look?

I've told other doctors to look for it, but **not one** of them saw it. How can that be? Am I hallucinating? Am I talking myself into seeing something that isn't true?

I obviously don't think so, or I wouldn't have gone to the trouble to write this book. When I first saw a patient respond to treatment after dairy products were eliminated from the diet, I was astounded. I actually didn't believe it until we manipulated the diet back and forth, first eliminating, then adding, then eliminating milk products again and again. It was as if we had found a switch with which we could turn symptoms on and then off again. I saw it enough in this first case to know that this patient experienced neck pain and back pain due to milk products, just like Robert Ester. "Wow," I thought, "he was right!" I assumed I had stumbled across another rare case of milk allergy causing musculoskeletal pain. I thought this discovery would help in those stubborn cases that did not respond to conventional chiropractic treatment.

That was six years ago. Since then, I have seen over 3000 different patients. I have seen the phenomenon over and over again, not just in a few cases, but **in the vast majority** of cases. This kind of study, my research, is what is called anecdotal, that is an accumulation of stories. Anecdotal research is usually discounted by the scientific community as unscientific, without proof or basis in fact. The incidence of lung cancer in smokers was an interesting anecdote for decades. The cigarette industry and doctors refuted these stories for years because there was no solid proof that cigarettes could be linked to lung cancer. So, scientists were forced to torture and kill countless laboratory animals, while people continued to die of lung cancer, before proof could be produced to the ultracritical scientific community. It wasn't until 1971 that the surgeon general made his official determination and placed his warning on cigarette packages.

The scientific community demands tests with controlled variables, using such statistical tools as control groups, placebos, double blind studies, etc. These tools supply evidence that either points to or refutes the hypothesis of the study. These tools are designed to eliminate all variables and isolate the one variable that is being tested. If patients recover from symptoms over a period of time, how do we know what got them better? How do we know if the patients or the researchers are reporting the truth? For example, if the subjects or the researchers know the hypothesis, they might tend to imagine symptoms that either support or dispute it. A double blind study is one in which the subjects and the researchers are not aware of what is being studied. A placebo is a preparation, or drug with little or no therapeutic value. In some studies that test the effectiveness of a certain drug, some subjects are given a placebo, because some of these people may imagine that there will be a change in symptoms just because they took a pill.

An anecdotal study does not use a laboratory setting, but rather the setting of real life. That's where patients live and experience symptoms. In real life. The real world. I'm a practitioner and see real patients. I don't have time to go into a lab and study the reactions of patients in a sterile, controlled environment just to satisfy closed minded doctors. The patients I see have even less time to play with their symptoms. You see, I'm interested in their symptoms. I want to study them, manipulate them, etc. But patients don't want to play with their symptoms. They just want them to go away and not come back.

The goal in my office is to determine the causes of symptoms in each case, then eliminate them so the patient can go on with his/her life without pain. I was taught in school that manipulation of the spine is a powerful tool in the management of cases of back pain and headaches. In the first few years of my practice, I used physical medicine in the management of these cases. My goal was to change the structure and mobility of the spine and the ligaments and muscles that affected it. I used manipulation, moist heat, electrical muscle stimulation, traction, and ultrasound to alleviate symptoms. This is physical medicine. I got fairly good results. I got conventional results. When I first began practicing chiropractic, I worked in a large sports medicine clinic. Working together in this clinic were chiropractors, massage therapists, a neurologist, an acupuncturist, and an acupressurist. Each and every patient was managed with a program of total health care. We gave them a list of exercises to perform at home and foods to eliminate from their diets. We treated all patients the same. We instructed all patients to eliminate sugar, salt, red meat, shell fish, alcohol, tobacco, caffeine, nicotine, and dairy products. A lot of patients were really bummed out. Actually, most of them didn't take us seriously. As the list got longer, I'm sure they thought, "he's got to be kidding." In addition to these changes, these patients were to come into the clinic multiple times for treatment, usually in a predetermined program, starting off at three times a week for a month, then two times a week for a month, then once a week for a month, then once a month for the rest of their lives, or until their insurance ran out. Most patients got better, and usually everyone, doctors and patients, believed that the real reason they got better was due to the spinal adjustments. Everyone could understand the relationship between the pain and the adjustment. The adjustment happened right where the pain was, and afterwards, the pain was decreased or gone. Immediately after the adjustment there was a noticeable increase in range of motion. We all assumed that changing the diet was designed solely to enhance the patient's overall health. That is, even though the patient came in to get rid of a particular complaint, we were also going to force them to get healthy. A healthy body will heal much faster and better than an unhealthy one.

We went one step further in managing these cases from a dietary point of view. We gave each patient a list of foods that produced acidity in the blood when ingested. They were instructed to avoid these foods.

The chemicals in the blood that cause inflammation at injury sights are mainly acidic. If the blood is more acidic due to acid producing foods in the diet, the inflammatory reaction to injury will be more acute, causing more pain. For example, if two identically conditioned athletes undergo the same amount of training in one day, the athlete with the more acidic blood will experience more muscle soreness. I think this is true.

As a young chiropractor just starting out in practice, I was certainly open to guidance and instruction. I was instructed to prescribe treatment as above. This seemed like a good way to practice, and it is, but I had my questions. I took over the practice of another chiropractor who was similarly instructed. He was about to move on, into his own practice. He trained me, and I asked him lots of questions. Like, why were patients instructed to avoid all these foods? The answers were as follows: Red meat, caffeine, and nicotine all caused the blood to become more acidic, increasing inflammation and therefor pain. Shellfish, like shrimp, lobster and scallops, are bad because they are highly allergenic foods. Dairy products were to be eliminated because they produce mucous.

People know that alcohol and tobacco are bad for them. After all, scientific studies have been performed. We know that alcohol and tobacco are bad. There are warnings on the packages, and in places where alcohol is served. We don't allow minors to use them, they cause bad things to happen to people, and eventually they kill you. People can live with that, though. "The world is going to hell, anyway!" or "You've gotta die of something!" We certainly didn't tell people to stop riding motorcycles without helmets. (Studies are inconclusive in that area.)

Most people, when told that dairy products produce mucous and phlegm, will clear their throats and say, "I can live with a little phlegm, just fix my pain, doc." Most people don't care that much about total health when they are experiencing excruciating headaches, or killer back pain, or any other acute condition. They want relief. Now.

That's why people prefer a pill that gives them instant relief if they can get one. When a doctor starts talking about a healthy lifestyle, many patients will interrupt and say, "that's great, doc, but isn't there a pill or a shot or an adjustment I can take to get rid of this pain right now?" Most people think there is no relationship between health and pain.

If a doctor tells them that their pain **may** be due to some food they love, like milk, they **might** eliminate it from their diets, but probably not. If the doctor expects a patient to change his/her diet, the doctor must convince the patient that there is definitely, not maybe, a correlation between their main complaint and what the doctor is telling them to do without. Then, the doctor has to let them know what to expect, how long it will take to see a change in symptoms. The patient can't wait around indefinitely for the pain to subside.

Once when I was giving a lay lecture, I asked if anyone had had back surgery, and did it help. One man raised his hand and said his surgery definitely helped, but he didn't see an improvement in his symptoms until four years after his surgery! I think he might have thought twice about going under the knife if the doctor had told him he would feel better in four years. Maybe not.

The purpose of this book is to describe my clinical experiences to illustrate that there is a definite connection between foods and symptoms, in this case, mainly between milk and dairy products and back pain and headaches. In order to establish this connection, the milk connection, several questions must be answered.

What physiological mechanism is at work when foods cause physical symptoms? What we are talking about here is food allergy. Now that is a very debatable issue, that is, whether the milk connection is actually an example of food allergy. Webster's defines **allergy** as "excess sensitivity producing a bodily reaction to certain substances as food, pollen, drugs, or heat or cold, which are harmless to most persons: common allergies are hay fever, hives, and asthma." An allergen is any substance that induces allergy. A **poison** is defined by Webster as "any agent that chemically destroys life or health upon contact with or absorption by an organism..."

Allergic reactions involve the immune system. An allergen affects **some** people in a bad way, people who, for some reason, are sensitive. Allergic reactions are not dose dependent. Quantity is not important. A little dab'll do ya, although some people are more sensitive than others. A poison affects **all** people in a bad way. Poisons are dose dependent. A little may make you sick, a lot will kill you.

Common allergies are common knowledge. When a person comes in contact with a plant, like poison ivy, and hives develop on the skin where contact was made, most people realize that an allergic reaction has taken place. When the plants bloom in spring, or you mow the lawn and all of a sudden start sneezing, you are usually easily convinced that an allergic reaction has occurred. Many people are aware that certain foods cause problems for them. Most medical questionnaires will ask patients to list any medications to which they are allergic. Many people are allergic to penicillin, for example.

What most people don't realize is that allergic reactions are not necessarily limited to skin reactions and respiratory symptoms. When a person eats a specific food and immediately gets a runny nose and eyes and sneezes, he or she usually suspects allergy. When they react in the same way to the same food several times, every time, they are usually convinced that they are allergic to that particular food. They also suspect that they

No Milk

will always react to that food each and every time they are exposed. If the allergic reaction is severe enough, most people are motivated to avoid eating that food in the future.

I know a woman who is allergic to cantaloupe. The last time she ate cantaloupe, her throat swelled shut, she became asphyxiated, and passed out. She had to be rushed to the hospital and nearly died. Fortunately, she recovered, and, even more fortunately, the doctors asked questions and determined that the cantaloupe was the culprit. Needless to say, she is highly motivated to avoid eating cantaloupe. She did not need multiple exposures to be convinced that she was allergic to cantaloupe. She doesn't even care if the doctors might be wrong. She doesn't want to find out. Her anecdotal study was sufficient for her. She can live fine, thank you very much, without cantaloupe. "How do you know?" doesn't motivate her at all.

I once saw a 65 year old female who had suffered with headaches her entire life. I treated her with chiropractic adjustments and instructed her to avoid all milk and dairy products. (I do not assume that all headaches are due to milk products. A thorough history made that treatment program my best guess.) After seven days her headaches were gone. She was released. I called her two months later to check on her progress.

"How are you doing?" I asked.

"Oh, okay I guess, but my headaches are back."

I was shocked. "I can't understand why."

"Oh, I can. I'm back on milk again."

"WHY???" I was incredulous.

"I guess I just love milk."

"So I guess you love milk more than hate your headaches?"

"I guess so."

At least she knew what caused her headaches and didn't need to consult doctors anymore. She just wasn't highly motivated to quit milk. **Almost all headaches are allergic reactions.** (Does "almost" mean 60%? 80%? No. About 99%!!)

But allergic reactions are many and varied. Allergy can manifest itself as joint and muscle pain, heart palpitations, drowsiness, mood changes, hyperactivity, muscle cramping, etc. Allergy can be any abnormality in the human condition. Allergy can cause antisocial behavior. Allergy can change your handwriting.

There. That ought to slam the door shut on a few closed minds.

However, if you're still in here reading along with an open mind, you've probably read some health magazines and probably already heard that. Figuring out allergy is difficult, because, not only are the symptoms many and varied, but so is the reaction time. An instantaneous reaction is the easiest to spot and accept, especially when the reaction is repeated several times. Mr. Ester reacted to milk with burning back pain when milk touched his lips — not when he swallowed it, not when the milk entered his stomach, not an hour or a day later, but **as it touched his lips.** After consulting so many physicians for his back pain, and never hearing mention of allergy to milk, he was shocked. He needed to repeat the experiment several times before he was convinced that milk was causing his back pain. But each time his reaction was consistent and instantaneous. Lucky for him and lucky for me. An instantaneous reaction is rare. Most reactions take anywhere from instantly to 48 hours to cause symptoms. Most allergic reactions to foods occur 2 to 12 hours after exposure. If Mr. Ester had the usual 12 hour reaction, he may not have made the milk connection.

What most doctors don't realize is that most disease is due to exposure to allergens or poisons. That's right, most disease. Earlier I mentioned that disease is caused by inherited weaknesses, trauma, exposure, and unknown causes.

The hospital rooms should be reserved for victims of trauma. Doctors need to be there to patch up the poor folks that have fallen off buildings, or have been burned, or have been run over by trucks.

No Milk

There will always be unknown causes, because what we know about the human body and disease is minimal compared to what we don't know. We need to sick the mavericks, the weirdos, the open minded creative thinkers into that arena, not the pharmaceutical companies. We have already figured out that we can cause almost anything or everything with drugs. But the chemistry of the body is an equation that must always be balanced. Drugs give something and take something. Look at Lyle Alzado. The steroids he took made him real big. The cancer they caused made him very small.

Inherited weaknesses should be dealt with by the doctors who study genetic traits and can prevent them with parental counseling. For a health care practitioner practicing in the trenches, trying to help sick people, considering inherited weaknesses is a waste of time. To charge a patient money to tell them that their problem "runs in the family" is not health care.

A distinction needs to be made here between **genetic traits and familial traits.** A genetic trait is one that is determined by genes, like blue eyes, tall stature, big hands, etc. Many people believe, or are told, that if their parents or uncles or siblings tend to have a particular health problem, they are likely to have it too. If back pain, or heart disease, or high blood pressure, or arthritis "runs in the family," many people cop to the notion that they deserve it too.

To establish specific locations on genes that represent specific traits is an exacting science. Scientists are studying the DNA in insects with the notion that once the locations of certain traits are established, we may be able to manipulate genetic traits in individuals. Don't hold your breath. Maybe some people with back pain or heart disease have specific genes that contribute to their illness. But to assume so with no proof is pointless. Most genetic traits cannot be changed.

Familial traits are those that occur in families due to similar habits. Evil Kneivel's son, Robbie, for example, didn't inherit weak bones. He just has the same habit as his father of crashing motorcycles for a living. If your father and your grandfather died of lung cancer, it doesn't mean it has been inherited and you are likely to get it. A closer look usually reveals a smoking habit, or jobs in coal mines. These examples seem silly just to illustrate a point. If a lot of your family members suffer with back pain, it doesn't necessarily mean that you will have back pain that can't be helped. Most people in this situation know that avoiding the heavy work of their forefathers does little to prevent back pain, so it must be genetic, right? No, almost never. Look to the diet.

Many American men want their new wives to cook like mom. That's why they end up looking like dad, back pain and all. The traits they seemingly "inherit" in many cases are familial, due to similar habits that have been passed down, and can be avoided by changing habits and lifestyles and diets.

Most people have little trouble being convinced that a family tendency for heart disease or high blood pressure could be caused by inherited dietary habits. Parents who use lots of salt teach their kids to acquire a taste for salt. Recipes and dietary habits are passed down. Even when people realize that heart disease runs in their family, seldom do they throw up their hands and "learn to live with it." Most doctors and patients realize that dietary changes can prevent a seemingly inevitable heart attack or bypass surgery.

But most doctors and patients fail to apply the same thinking to cases of back pain, headaches, or arthritis. For a doctor to perform expensive tests that offer no hope or change in a treatment program, then prescribe lifetime medication and the advice to "learn to live with pain" until the inevitable surgery is performed, is an impotent treatment program. A doctor must offer some hope in every case, some course of action. If he paints a picture of gloom and doom and "there's nothing that can be done," he's not a health care practitioner. He's just a medicine man.

In my opinion, the most hopeless diagnoses in medicine today is arthritis. A patient with joint pain consults the doctor. The doctor performs a battery of tests — gosh, he's so thorough. Blood tests, x-rays, CT scans. He leaves no rock unturned. When the testing is done, the patient waits for the doctor with bated breath. The doctor gathers up all the evidence and takes it into the room with the patient. The patient shivers with anticipation.

"What is it, doc? Did you find anything."

"Yep. It's arthritis."

As a chiropractor, most of my patients complain of some sort of musculoskeletal pain. Many of these people have been to their medical doctors first. Most of them who are over 40 have been diagnosed as having arthritis. Arthritis, like most seemingly complex medical words, is Latin: Arth = joint, and itis = inflammation. So tonsillitis is inflammation of the tonsils, tendinitis is inflammation of the tendons, and arthritis is inflammation of the joints.

The American public has come to assume that arthritis is inevitable, something we all get eventually and just can't help. So, when the x-rays have all been taken, and the blood tests come back, and the patient is waiting in the treatment room (forever) with bated breath, the doctor gathers the evidence, comes in and says, "Well, it's arthritis."

Out comes that bated breath, a sigh of relief, surrender.

"Take this medication forever and learn to live with the pain."

People actually pay for that.

Let me tell you folks, arthritis does cause pain, and is responsible for the pain that some people experience. Arthritis is visible on an x-ray film. But the fact is, **x-ray is an overrated diagnostic tool.** When the area of complaint is x-rayed, anything abnormal that shows up on the film is presumed to be the cause of the problem. Many people, doctors and patients, believe that the answer is somewhere on that black and white film. That is a huge assumption. Everyone stares at the film. The doctor is searching for something, anything abnormal. When arthritis shows up on the film, the doctor will usually stop his search for the cause of the problem, and so will the patient. Many people stop their search for help when they hear that magic word and rely on medication for life.

* If arthritis is indeed the problem, why does the patient have arthritis? Some people suffer with severe arthritis in their twenties. Many seventy year-old Americans suffer with arthritis, but a lot of them don't. Why does one person have it, yet another doesn't? What is the cause of arthritis? (I know, it runs in your family). Believe me, arthritis is not inevitable. If it is there, something caused it.

There are two main kinds of arthritis: osteoarthritis, or degenerative, and rheumatoid arthritis. Osteoarthritis develops usually as a result of wear and tear on joints and bones. It is visible on x-rays and is usually described as "lipping and spurring," or "DJD (Degenerative Joint Disease)." After multiple traumas to a joint, the synovial membranes, or soft tissue component of the joints, start to wear out, putting increased pressure on the bony surfaces. The bones then adapt to the stress by increasing their bony supports with lips and spurs (osteophytes). The joint surfaces of the bones increase in calcification and appear whiter on x-ray. Many times, the ligaments around the joint calcify. Eventually, as the soft tissue between the bones wears out, the bones end up closely approximated as movement in the joint becomes more and more difficult and limited. If the person survives long enough, the joint will become fused, and movement will cease all together.

Rheumatoid arthritis is an inflammation of the soft tissues of the joint. Inflammation means heat, redness, and swelling. The joints are swollen and tender and painful to move. Cases range in severity from moderate occasional pains, to severe swelling and degenerative changes that totally disable the patient from any kind of normal functioning. A joint is a blood tight capsule that exists between two bones. A thin membrane lines the ends of the bones. The joint capsule contains a fluid that acts as a lubricant between the bones and allows fluid movement. In rheumatoid arthritis, the membranes become inflamed and thicken. The joints appear swollen, red, and painful. The finger joints are easily visible as they are not covered by overlying muscle. (The muscles that move the fingers are stored in the forearms). Rheumatoid arthritis of the knuckles can be very deforming. Other joints, especially the many joints of the spine, are covered with many layers of muscles, and arthritis pain here is not so graphic.

Most doctors who don't specialize in spinal diagnosis and care will diagnose any kind of chronic back pain as arthritis. The fact is, arthritis is usually only one of the descriptive symptoms that describes the physical condition of a joint or joints. For some reason, everyone, doctor, patient, and family, nods knowingly and says, "I told you" when they hear that magic word. They feel as smart as the doctor. They may or may not be as smart, but they can do as much as the doctor can. They don't have any drug samples in their desk drawers, but over-the-counter pain remedies are as good as prescription drugs. The main difference between prescription drugs and over-the-counter drugs is the side effects. The theory is that the doctor can warn the patient before he gives them a prescription drug.

Many people believe that the pharmaceutical companies are going to come up with a pill that will "cure" arthritis. I've got some bad news for them, and all doctors must one day learn this: The only way to cure disease and stop symptoms is to determine the cause of the symptoms and eliminate it. Period. There will never be a pill that cures arthritis. There will never be a pill that cures cancer. There will never be a pill that cures heart disease. There will never be a pill that a fighter can take before he steps into the ring with Mike Tyson that will keep him from getting knocked out.

So, it must necessarily follow: What is the cause of arthritis? Let's look it up. *Taber's Medical Dictionary* says, "Arthritis may result from or be associated with a number of conditions including: infection (gonoccocal, tuberculous, pneumococcal); rheumatic fever; ulcerative colitis; trauma; neurogenic disturbances; degenerative joint disease as osteoarthritis; metabolic disturbances as gout; neoplasms [that bad word, CANCER]; hydrarthrosis; para or periarticular conditions as fibromyositis, myositis, or bursitis; various other conditions as acromegaly, psoriasis, Raynaud's Disease."

Makes you want to sit down and read a medical dictionary, doesn't it? So what does all that mean? All those "itis's" and other conditions suggest other systems that are breaking down in conjunction with the joint breakdown of arthritis. So does ulcerative colitis cause arthritis, or vice versa?

I would like to make a smooth progression through this text to the point of the book, but this definition from *Taber's* is useful in illustrating a point that will occur later in the book, and that has to do with multiple system involvement in the disease process.

In clinical diagnosis we are taught that patients who suffer with ulcerative colitis often suffer with arthritis. The causal relationship between the two is not discussed in medical texts, just something to help the doctor arrive at that all-important Latin or Greek name tag, the diagnosis. Let's describe the patient's complaints and translate them into Latin. So if you have severe abdominal discomfort, gas and bloating, and your joints hurt, we have a name for that: Ulcerative colitis.

Once the diagnosis is made, that foreign word is the entry key into the conventional medicine computer. Punch the key, up comes the treatment program, in this case, anti-inflammatory drugs for the joint pain, and a bland diet to help soothe the ulcerative colitis (inflammation of the colon). When the disease progresses to the point of blood and pus in the stool, remove the colon and attach an external bag to the patient. Possibly psychotherapy to help the patient deal with the bag and the family and the public, etc.

But amazingly enough, the main cause of ulcerative colitis is also the main cause of arthritis. What is it? What's the title of this book?

Conventional medical wisdom disagrees: Medical textbooks mention that dairy products should be limited. At the same time, however, they say, "Although a role of diet in ulcer causation is often hypothesized, there is no direct evidence to incriminate either particular diets or elements of diets such as hot spices."[1]

Medics think diet is not important. I think diet is all-important.

One of us is dead wrong.

So, if an infection is causing a joint to swell, kill the infection. If you sprained your finger playing softball, use ice for the swelling, let it heal, and try not to do it again. There's no pill for that. If a metabolic disorder, such as gout, is causing the problem, fix it. Gout is a malfunctioning in the body's ability to breakdown purines. Purines are in high concentration in meat and booze. When the body can't break them down, uric acid accumulates and crystalizes in a joint, or several joints, and causes severe inflammation and pain. You can take a pill if you want, but it only makes sense, once you know what the doctor knows, to stop eating meat and drinking booze.

So, what if you don't drink booze or eat meat, you don't play softball, and you really can't remember doing anything to deserve your pain, but the doctor says your problem is arthritis? First of all, maybe it's not arthritis. But let's assume it is. Most medical people will answer that arthritis is inherited, or that the causes are unknown. I have a simple mind, and when I see a patient complain of symptoms that occur all over the body, I look for a cause that is in the blood. Rarely does any trauma or activity cause symptoms all over the body. Blood carries its products everywhere in the human body. Nutrients taken into the body are metabolized in the intestines, then either excreted or absorbed into the blood for transport to all the tissues of the body. The blood is composed of chemicals that have been ingested or inhaled. For the cause of symptoms that occur throughout the body, look first to the diet. This book is about milk and back pain, but, if you experience wide ranging symptoms, no matter what they are, **look to the diet.**

---

[1] James Wingaarden, *Cecil Textbook of Medicine* (W.B. Saunders, 1982).

An old M.D. once wrote a book about arthritis. He said that the cause of arthritis is the three white evils. I say there are four white evils, the three he named: sugar, salt, and bleached flour. The fourth is milk. I believe milk is the worst of the white evils. I also believe it causes arthritis in many people. These four white evils cause all kinds of problems in the human body, one of them is arthritis. There are many other foods that, in some people, cause arthritis and other problems. Food sensitivities and allergies are more common than most doctors realize, and the symptoms they cause are many and varied.

When a doctor says you have arthritis, let the questioning begin. Don't give up. Don't resign yourself to medication. Don't learn to live with your pain until you have asked all the questions, until you have asked other sufferers, until you have asked multiple health care professionals, until you have cleaned up your diet, **until you die!**

So, I believe that back pain or headaches caused by the ingestion of milk products is an example of an allergic reaction. Most allergies are due to repeated exposure to specific substances. For some reason, the overly exposed system reacts by building an immune system that is specific for a certain allergen. Specialized T cells and lymphocytes are built and programmed to identify the specific allergen. These specialized cells line the mucous membranes of the digestive tract, the respiratory tract, the blood vessels, and the organ systems throughout the body. They are programmed to identify, then attack a specific protein structure, like the protein of penicillin, or that of bee venom, or one of the proteins in cow's milk.

No one experiences an allergic reaction to an allergen on the first exposure. No one has an allergic reaction to their first dose of penicillin. The immune system must first "see" the protein structure of the allergen one or several times before it can build the specialized cells that will attack upon future exposure. Some people can take penicillin for years, then all of a sudden become allergic to it. Some people can drink cow's milk for a lifetime and never develop an allergy to it. Some infants develop allergy to cow's milk when their only exposure is to mom's milk when she has been drinking cow's milk. The milk protein passes from mom, to mom's milk, to the nursing infant. A nursing baby can also develop an allergy to penicillin by nursing on mom, who has been drinking cow's milk from a cow that was treated with penicillin. Penicillin passed from the cow, to its milk, to mom, to her milk, to the baby. We don't know why an allergy all of a sudden develops. Our lack of understanding of the details of allergy and its mechanisms cause rigid scientists to doubt this kind of work.

When I was in college in Southern California, I bought two Siamese cats. I lived with them in the house for four years. I could pet them, sleep with them, and cuddle them for hours with no negative reactions. When I graduated, I moved to Phoenix to attend graduate school. Within a few weeks I began waking up each night with a severe cough. After several months of this, I went to the doctor. I figured I had contacted some virus that was indigenous to Arizona, like Valley Fever. The doctor told me I had bronchitis, cause unknown. After one year of this misery, I was forced to give the cats away (My ex-wife won the custody battle). My night time coughs stopped, although I didn't realize it at the time.

That's a funny thing about human nature. I've seen patients who suffer with a complaint for years, and when it goes away they don't even notice. It has to be pointed out to them. We seem to have a short memory for pain. I think that's why some women have several children.

Anyway, after a year or so with no cough, I acquired a new kitten. My night coughs began immediately and I realized my cough was an allergic reaction to cats. My little story here (true, by the way) is an example of a positive test for allergy. It wasn't done in a lab, it's an anecdote, a story — hardly scientific. But the story follows the basic rules of allergy testing. There is only one accurate way to test for allergy:

(1) Expose patient to allergen and observe symptoms.

(2) Remove allergen and observe symptoms stop.

(3) Re-expose patient to allergen and observe a return of symptoms.

Conventional allergists, who practice conventional medicine, do not use this testing method. There are two kinds of allergists practicing today: Conventional allergists, and bio-ecologists (also called clinical ecologists). The testing method described above is used by bio-ecologists, practitioners who study the reaction of the human organism to the environment. Those of us who practice bio-ecology realize that most disease is due to exposure to allergens and/or poisons through inhalation, direct contact, inoculation, or ingestion.

Conventional allergists are the allies of conventional medicine. They like to get complex and scientific. They test for allergy using a skin or blood test. This testing is not accurate or repeatable. Most patients who consult a conventional allergist find out they are allergic to pollens, molds, dust, animal dander, and some foods. It seems they all get the same list. Since avoiding all of these allergens is next to impossible, a treatment program of years of allergy shots is recommended. The results are poor.

Bio-ecologists are the doctors that treat disease caused by exposure to allergens and/or poisons. Most disease is due to exposure, but sadly, most patients are consulting conventional practitioners who think, and tell their patients that the rest of us are wrong, or nuts. These conventional practitioners seem to believe that most disease is due to a lack of some medication. Conventional chiropractors seem to believe that chronic pain calls for chronic treatment.

After my encounter with Robert Ester, and my clinical experiences of the last six years, I have become what I call a chiropractic bio-ecologist. Medical bio-ecologists, like Dr. Marshall Mandell and Dr. Robert Foreman, realize that most disease is due to exposure to allergens or poisons. As a chiropractor, I have come to realize that most cases of back pain, neck pain, and/or headaches are due to exposure to allergens and/or poisons.

No Milk

In my clinical experience, I have seen that virtually any allergen that produces a reaction in a sensitive person, can cause virtually any symptom. I have seen patients who experienced neck pain, back pain, and/or headaches due to exposure to tomatoes, squash, wheat, and soy. I will discuss many reactions in the story section, but here I will deal with the biggy — milk and dairy products.

MILK AND DAIRY PRODUCTS

Dairy products include all foods made with or from cow's milk. Although eggs are found in the dairy section at the grocery, they are not considered dairy products. Of course, milk is from a cow, eggs are from chickens. Cow's milk is made of a solid component, curd, and a liquid component, whey. (Yes, Little Miss Muffet sat on her tuffet, eating her cottage cheese). Like all "perfect" foods, milk is made up of carbohydrates, fats, and proteins. Cow's milk contains about 4.9% carbohydrate in the form of lactose, the milk sugar, 3.5 to 4.4% fat, and 3.5 to 3.8% protein. Minerals and other substances make up about 0.7%. The remaining 87% is water.

Lactose, the milk sugar, is found in cow's milk and in human milk. Lactose consists of two sugars, glucose and galactose. In order for us to utilize these sugars as energy sources, they must be broken apart and absorbed. That task is accomplished in the small intestines by an enzyme called lactase. Humans have the highest concentration of lactase in the intestines immediately after birth. This is by design, of course, so the nursing infant can break down and utilize the lactose in mom's milk. As the human infant grows and develops, the concentration of lactase naturally decreases until the infant loses the desire to nurse. This takes about 12 to 18 months. So, by design, the human infant should be sustained only on mom's milk until the infant decides on his or her own to stop. That is what Nature has designed, but what society and modern medicine have redesigned for convenience.

As the human infant is naturally weaned from breast milk, the concentration of lactase diminishes and, along with it, the ability to digest lactose. When lactose cannot be broken down into glucose and galactose, it cannot be absorbed. If lactose continues to be dumped into the intestine without sufficient lactase, it accumulates and ferments, causing gas and bloating and diarrhea. Nature is aware of this, so Nature tells the infant to stop nursing.

Unfortunately, Nature has not given the infant enough size and strength to smack mom when she carries him or her out to the pasture to start nursing on some barn yard animal, like a cow. When the lactose from cow's milk starts accumulating in the poor little infant's intestines, all he or she can do is fart and cry, hoping mom will pull her off the udder.

The inability to digest lactose is called lactose intolerance. Not all humans suffer from lactose intolerance, just most of them. Not all people drink cow's milk. Some people maintain enough lactase in the intestines to successfully digest cow's milk. Some people think gas and diarrhea and indigestion are normal.

Most people in this country have become aware that heart disease is a major problem here, and largely due to fat and cholesterol in the diet. Cow's milk is high in fat and cholesterol. The dairy industry has addressed this issue by producing low fat, non fat, 1% fat, 2% fat, and skim milk products. The mentality of most health conscious people has motivated them to "cut back" on their dairy products, or to use skim milk or low fat milk. However, milk remains a vital part of their diet so they can get their calcium, one of the essential minerals in milk that make it such a supposedly great health food.

The minerals in milk are calcium, phosphorus, iron, sodium, and potassium. Most people are motivated to drink milk for the essential calcium. American women have been indoctrinated to fear osteoporosis, brittle bone disease caused presumably by calcium deficiency. The thinking is, that by increasing dietary calcium, the bones will become stronger and osteoporosis will be avoided. This has become common knowledge.

Beware of common knowledge.

No Milk

The AMA (American Medical Association) and the dairy industry in this country have determined that we need 1000 to 1500 milligrams of dietary calcium per day to maintain optimum health. The best source of dietary calcium, they claim, is milk and dairy products.

Asian and African people do not consume milk and have a daily calcium intake of less than 400 milligrams a day, yet they have healthy teeth and do not suffer from osteoporosis. The assumption is that calcium in the diet will be absorbed and utilized by the body. Calcium metabolism is not that simple. The absorption rate of calcium is dependent upon, for one thing, its ratio to dietary phosphorus. Phosphorus can combine with calcium in the intestines and prevent the absorption of calcium. For ideal calcium absorption, the source should contain a ratio of calcium to phosphorus of 2:1. The calcium/phosphorus ratio in cow's milk is 1:1, making cow's milk a poor source of dietary calcium. Cow's milk has 1200 milligrams of calcium per quart, whereas human milk has only 300 milligrams of calcium per quart, yet infants absorb more calcium due to the calcium to phosphorus ratio, which is nearly 2:1 in human milk.

The absorption of calcium is also affected by the amount of protein in the diet. When a high protein diet is consumed, the excess protein is broken down in the liver and excreted through the kidneys. When proteins are broken down, they show up in the blood as blood urea nitrogen (BUN). Urea in the blood has a diuretic effect, causing the kidneys to excrete more water. Along with the water, calcium is excreted in the urine. Cow's milk is a high protein food.

Five of the top meat and dairy users in the world are the United States, Finland, Israel, England, and Sweden. These countries also have the highest incidence of osteoporosis in the world. So the idea of using a high dairy intake to prevent osteoporosis is not working.

Contrary to what you have been told, cow's milk is a poor source of calcium. Although the concentration of calcium in milk is high, it is poorly absorbed. Drinking milk for calcium makes about as much sense as smoking for weight control.

The facts about calcium are these: humans can get all the calcium they need for optimum health from a normal diet of vegetables, fruits, rice, and beans. Cows produce lots of calcium without drinking milk. Cows are vegetarians. **Calcium deficiency of dietary origin is unknown in humans.**

The protein in cow's milk consists mainly of:

casein
lactoalbumin
lactoglobulin

Approximately 77% of the protein in cow's milk is casein. Milk consists of curd, the solid part, and whey, the liquid part. When cheese is made, the curd makes up the cheese, and the milk serum, the whey, is the byproduct, not part of the cheese. So cheese contains the casein and not the other two proteins, lactoalbumin and lactoglobulin.

When I first noticed the milk connection, I saw that patients who were sensitive, reacted to milk, cheese, ice cream, sour cream, etc. That is, they reacted to all foods made with cow's milk. I knew that whey was also a product of cow's milk, so, being thorough, I instructed patients to also avoid whey. Whey is used in many packaged foods, like breads and margarine. Eliminating butter and margarine severely limited the average diet. Avoiding all dairy products and reading labels looking for whey became a monumental task for most patients. After some patients became aware of their reactions, some informed me that they did not react to whey. After I heard this several times, I decided to remove whey from the list of foods to be avoided. Over the years, I have had only one patient report to me that he reacted to whey. All other patients who are sensitive to milk and dairy products have reported no reaction to whey.

Since allergy is a reaction to specific proteins, this has lead me to believe that the aggravating agent, or allergen, in cow's milk is casein. Since most people are aware that dairy products are unhealthy because of their high fat content, they have made an attempt to improve their health by changing from whole milk to low fat, or skim milk, or non-fat milk. Many men relate to me that their wives have them on that "watered down stuff." Even medical doctors who don't have any nutritional training suggest to patients that low fat is better than whole milk. And this is true.

When asked about their use of dairy products, many patients will point out that they only use non-fat milk, or "only" non-fat milk. That's good, as far as limiting dietary fat. But when the patient suffers from back pain, neck pain, joint pain, or headaches due to allergy to milk, the fat content is not a factor. The milk protein, casein, is in non-fat as well as whole milk. The allergic reaction can be avoided only if all dairy products containing casein are totally avoided.

• Many patients are aware that they suffer digestive distress when they drink milk. They get gas and bloating, or diarrhea. Some people throw up any milk they drink. This is lactose intolerance, an inability to digest lactose, the milk sugar. Most Americans are aware of this disorder because it is common, and the dairy industry has dealt with it by developing commercial products such as Lactaid™ milk and Lactaid™ tablets. Lactaid™ milk is low in lactose, so is more easily tolerated by people with low concentrations of lactase, the enzyme necessary to break down the milk sugar. Lactaid™ tablets can be taken with dairy products to help in digestion, and to limit the gas and other symptoms people experience with lactose intolerance. Again, milk allergy will not be affected by Lactaid™ products. The casein is the problem, and is still present in these products.

It amazes me that milk is still considered the "perfect food." The dairy industry is pushing new products because the fat content of their "perfect food" is too high and is one of the main contributors to heart disease, the number one health problem in our country. They want people who throw up milk or get stomach cramps to keep drinking the stuff by taking a pill after each dose.

The dairy industry and other social pressures have convinced mothers to pull their newborns from their breasts at earlier and earlier ages so mom can get on with a job, or life, or just away from the baby. At first moms were convinced to go right to the bottle with cow's milk. Now infant formula has been inserted between breast feeding and the onslaught of cow's milk because so many babies couldn't tolerate cow's milk. Human milk is 80% whey and 20% casein. Cow's milk is just the opposite. Manufacturers are now producing formula that is more like mom's milk than cow's milk, that is, whey predominant. But most Americans "know" that eventually, no matter how their children feel, or act, or complain, or don't complain, cow's milk, that perfect food, absolutely **must** become part of the diet. Wrong, wrong, wrong, wrong, wrong.

The dairy industry, and some of the health care practitioners and politicians they have in their pockets, have so successfully brainwashed the American public that cow's milk is good, even necessary, that we feel obligated to go through all these charades just to get the stuff down! I don't understand this mentality. It makes about as much sense as filters on cigarettes, or lean meat!

But the point here is that milk allergy is unaffected by products that attempt to deal with the milk fat and the milk sugar. The problem is the protein, casein. More and more doctors are becoming aware that the number one food allergy is cow's milk. As this knowledge filters into the public, and milk sales start to drop, I'm sure the dairy industry will develop a low protein version of their "perfect food" for adults.

Americans will eventually realize that the fat of cow's milk, the sugar of cow's milk, and the protein of cow's milk should be eliminated. They must realize that the antibiotics and steroids that the cow is exposed to will show up in the milk. Hopefully, they will come to the obvious conclusion that cow's milk should be eliminated all together. But for now, to avoid the physical symptoms of milk allergy, the protein, casein, must be avoided all together.

No Milk

Casein is found in the following foods:

milk	ice milk	chocolate
cheese	sherbet	
cream cheese	whipped cream	
cottage cheese	sour cream	
cheese food	yogurt	
ice cream	butter	

Many doctors have suspected that headaches and other allergy symptoms are aggravated by certain dairy products. However, they demonstrate their lack of understanding of allergy by their treatment programs. I have had patients tell me that doctors suspected dairy products and instructed them to "cut back" on their use of milk products.

There are two problems with this advice. First of all, if a person is sensitive, or allergic to a certain substance, **any** exposure will cause a reaction. Once the immune system has become sensitive to a certain protein (allergic), the system will respond when any amount of that specific protein is ingested. Many people wear "Medic Alert" wrist bands alerting medical personnel to drug allergies, like penicillin or sulfa drugs. The warning doesn't say, "Allergic to penicillin — use only a little bit." These people and doctors realize that a little bit of penicillin will cause a reaction. People who are allergic to bee stings know that even a little bee will cause a reaction. The only way to avoid a reaction is to avoid any and all exposure. An allergic reaction is not dose dependent. This rule applies to allergy to dairy products.

The other problem with advising a patient to "cut back on milk products" is the lack of an explanation about what "milk products" are. I have been analyzing peoples' diets for years. I have learned many techniques to get an accurate accounting of a patient's dietary habits. After six years I still miss a lot. I have read my notes on patients I saw six years ago. It embarrasses me.

I used to ask patients if they used dairy products. If they responded "no" or "very little" I would move on, considering that a reaction to dairy products was not a factor in their case. As I became more experienced, I became more thorough. I have now moved well past thoroughness and am now considered relentless. Relentless questioning will still leave plenty of uncovered ground. But being relentless often leads to the truth. In fact, in most cases, relentless questioning is the only road to the truth, the whole truth, and nothing but the truth. I think that's why my chiropractic friends have discounted my work. You not only have to look to see the truth, but, in some cases, you have to look hard.

Now, when a patient says he or she doesn't use dairy products, I proceed to more specific questions. These questions are designed for several reasons:

To establish general dietary habits.

To establish the frequency and use of dairy products (exposure)

To look for other possible allergens or poisons.

My line of questioning moves from topic to topic, so the patient doesn't see a trend, try to guess what I'm after, and consequently slant his or her answers so they are "right". I want random answers, like what comes to mind first.

My first question usually is:

"Do you drink coffee?"

Most American adults answer that they do.

"How much?"

"Two or three cups. Only in the morning."

"Do you drink it black?"

"No. Cream and sugar."

"Do you eat breakfast?"

"Yes, just a bowl of cereal."

"Do you use milk on your cereal?"

"Yeah, just a dash of low fat."

"How often do you eat cereal."

"Only once a day."

"Every day?"

"Except on weekends, then I have eggs or pancakes."

Now, we have discovered that this person who initially reports that he or she doesn't use dairy products, uses some every day. And we haven't even made it past breakfast. I then proceed to lunch and dinner, asking the patient to describe typical meals. I ask if they snack during the day, do they eat out, or at home. What do they drink? Are there any foods they are allergic to? Are there any foods they crave?

The answers to these questions give only a general guideline as to the patient's dietary habits. To get a true picture of the patient's diet, I have to listen very closely before a dietary connection can be established or discounted. You see, I'm relentless because, in chronic cases, I believe there is **always** a dietary connection. Always, always, always!

Yes, it's true, I'm a fanatic.

Always?

Yes always.

"Do you always find the dietary connection?"

Unfortunately, no. But that doesn't mean it's not there.

Despite being relentless and thorough, the way I practice is very inaccurate. I rely on the memory of the patient and the honesty of the patient. I can't go home with the patients. These are very shady areas in most people, and that's not a put down. Who thinks about what they ate? To get to the truth, I rely on lots of tools. One of them is relentless questioning.

After asking general questions about the diet, I get more specific.

"Do you eat cheese?"

"Yes."

"How often in an average week?"

"Only about once a week, if that."

Now, that could be true, but the average American eats more cheese than that. So if I get an answer like this, I will clarify:

"I mean cheese on sandwiches, in salads, in Mexican food, pizza...?"

This will usually prompt the patient to recall a more accurate accounting of his or her diet, but not always. This is in no way an implication that patients lie. Most people are just not aware of what they eat. Relentless questioning, short of badgering, will help the patient begin to get an awareness of his or her diet. Badgering will usually chase the patient into a shell and cause the dietary information to be useless. Badgering also implies that the interrogator is leading the patient. The truth is always there, and will usually become apparent without creating data.

To establish a patient's use of dairy products, I ask about each item separately and how often, in an average week, they consume each item: ice cream, sour cream, yogurt, cottage cheese, etc. The average American uses dairy products regularly. When patients convey to me that they seldom use these products, even more specific questions are required. Sometimes, just a spot check of a specific meal is revealing. "What did you have for dinner last night?"

"Pizza."

Okay, they hardly ever have cheese, but they just happened to eat some last night. It could happen. At this point, there is no need to doubt a patient's accounting of his or her dietary habits. When a sincere patient reports to me little or no use of dairy products in the diet, I usually say, "Good, then it will be easy for you to avoid them."

Almost always, these patients return for subsequent visits and say, "You know, I didn't realize how often I use dairy products until I tried to avoid them. It seems every time I reached for something in the fridge, or planned a meal, I was using cheese, or milk, or sour cream." That's because that is the average American diet, the cause of average American health.

No Milk

More and more I see patients who have made an attempt to cut back on unhealthy food, and many of them realize that dairy products should be limited. But "limited" means different things to different people.

I saw a patient recently that I hadn't seen for a year. I had previously indoctrinated him about milk products. So, I asked him about his current use of dairy products.

"Minimal. Almost none", he responded.

I used to let that slide, but not now.

"How much milk are you drinking?"

"Only a glass a day, and it's skim milk."

That, ladies and gentleman, is not **heavy** use ... that is **regular** use. Again, allergic reactions are not dose dependent. Quantity is not the important factor, but regularity of exposure is. I have seen patients who drink a gallon of milk a day, and that's not uncommon. That, is **heavy** exposure. I have seen patients who have ice cream every night, plus some milk and cheese almost every day. And that's not uncommon. That is **heavy** exposure. I have seen patients who eat chocolate every day. They are usually women, by the way. That, is **heavy** exposure. (More on chocolate later).

To have **regular** exposure, all that is necessary is exposure every three days. A typical reaction to one exposure lasts three to four days. If a patient is sensitive to casein, and has some **only** a couple times a week, he or she could suffer constant symptoms, like headache, or back pain, or joint pain or stiffness, or lethargy, or irritability, **all the time.**

So, if a person has a little cheese on Monday, and some milk on cereal on Thursday, and some buttermilk pancakes on the weekend, and no other dairy products, they could have constant symptoms that doctors have told them is chronic. If they are sensitive to casein.

Not everyone is sensitive, or allergic to dairy products. Some people, believe it or not, can drink lots of milk their entire lives, and never have a single health problem as a result. That is, not a noticeable health problem. I'm often asked if everyone has problems with milk. Well, no, I don't think so, but I really don't know. I don't see people who don't have health problems. "Gee doc, I'm feeling great, just have some extra cash and want to get checked out." That doesn't happen to me. I don't think cow's milk is good food. I think it's unhealthy. But, not everyone is allergic to it. But I think many people have health problems due to the use of dairy products, health problems that are not noticeable, or that they don't relate as health problems. Most people don't know how good they can feel, or how good they are supposed to feel. Many people think they are "healthy as a horse" until they keel over at age 53, or have a stroke at age 77, or develop arthritis or Parkinson's Disease. Many people think "getting old" means being tired, or stiff, or slow, or boring. They think that's normal. I don't.

Americans have become used to so many "goodies" as a regular part of life, that they don't want to give them up. Sure, we all know people who smoke a pack a day, or drink a pint of whisky a day, or participate in some unhealthy activity, but are still spry and going strong at 95. Good for them. If Americans think that that's living, and some do, then so be it. But to participate in this sort of a lifestyle with the hopes that your luck will be the same is like playing the lottery for a living. Good luck.

To avoid casein means to not only avoid all milk products, but all foods made with milk. All of a sudden, the chore becomes more difficult. Robert Ester told me a story about his sensitivity to milk:

"One Sunday, my wife and I were out for an early morning drive. We pulled into a donut store to get some donuts to take home and have with coffee. She chose one, and so did I. I asked the man behind the counter if mine was made with milk. He said 'no.' We took the donuts home and made a pot of coffee. I took one bite of my donut and instantly got a headache and shooting pain in my spine. I wrapped up the rest of the donut, and the following day took it back to the donut store. A different man was behind the counter. I showed him the donut and informed him that I had been told on Sunday that it did not contain milk, and could he verify that. He apologized for the misinformation and said that the manufacturer had just recently changed the batter mix, and it now included non fat dry milk. That", he said, "is how sensitive I am to milk."

The following list is foods that are commonly made with milk:

pancakes	biscuits
waffles	ranch dressing
french toast	bleu cheese dressing
omelettes	some breads
mashed potatoes	most donuts
gravy	pizza

This list could go on and on, but the idea is, many foods are made with milk, and any exposure can cause symptoms in people who are allergic or sensitive to casein. Eating in restaurants, or at other people's houses is risky business.

"Gee, this is so hard," many people say.

Yes, it is, I guess, but it gets worse.

Many products are labelled "non-dairy." Man's best attempts to duplicate the taste of cow's milk are poor at best. Most milk substitutes are derived from soy, and if you've tried any of them, you can be sure you are not drinking cow's milk. Manufacturers of non-dairy items will often fudge a little bit to make their products taste more like cow's milk. They do this by adding an ingredient that will appear on the label as "sodium caseinate" or "calcium caseinate". Many times the manufacturer will actually mention that this additive is from cow's milk by labelling "sodium caseinate (a milk derivative)." A person who is allergic to casein will also react to sodium or calcium caseinate.

This additive also appears in some diet foods to add taste. Many people consider that mayonnaise is made with milk, I guess because it's white and creamy. But most mayonnaise is made with eggs and oil. Again, eggs are not dairy products, they are from chickens, not cows. However, diet, or low calorie mayonnaise is usually enhanced with sodium caseinate. "Miracle Whip™ Lite Mayonnaise" is an example. A person who is allergic to casein will react to these products.

I used to omit coffee in my dietary questioning, and of course, many people use cream and or sugar in their coffee. Many people who know they are allergic to milk, use milk in their coffee every day. This again, is regular exposure and will cause problems. Black coffee has a unique, very bitter taste, that many people don't like, but they enjoy the coffee flavor when the bitterness is dulled with cream. Many people have found that the powdered non-dairy creamers are cheaper, more convenient, and will still modify the taste of coffee to their liking. They also figure that a powdered non-dairy creamer is not milk and so can be used in a milk free diet. Sorry. Cremora™, Coffeemate™, Von's™, and every other brand I have seen, use sodium caseinate to give their product that milk flavor.

There are many liquid forms of non-dairy creamers on the market, however, most of them use sodium caseinate to enhance the flavor and simulate real milk. Mocha Mix™ is one that is made from soy milk that does not use sodium caseinate, or any form of the milk protein. So Mocha Mix™ is a viable substitute for milk and will not cause milk allergy symptoms. (However, it will cause symptoms if you are allergic to soy, which is one of the top five food allergies). Mocha Mix™ can be used as a coffee creamer, or as "milk" on cereal, or used in recipes that call for milk. The carton contains information on how to use it. Mocha mix is thick and creamy, like half and half, so it may be more palatable if diluted with water 2:1, or 3:1, or to taste.

The following list includes some foods that contain sodium caseinate:

Coffeemate™ non-dairy creamer
Cremora™
Miracle Whip™ Lite
Slim Fast™
Ultra Slim Fast™

Butter is, of course, made from milk and includes casein, so will therefor cause allergic symptoms. Most Americans are in the habit of buttering their bread, or potatoes, or vegetables, or whatever will take it. Most of them with heart problems have been instructed to switch to margarine because of the lower fat. Most margarine is made with whey, the by-product of cheese that contains the other two milk proteins, lactoalbumin and lactoglobulin. As I have said, I have seen, or had reported to me, only one patient who claimed he reacted to whey with similar symptoms. We must remember that a person can be allergic to anything, and patients must always consider that they may react to one or both of these proteins. Also, maybe I'm wrong about the aggravating agent being casein. Maybe it's some other additive, or chemical, or something in milk that causes the reactions. Going back again to the premise of this book, all I know for sure is that many patients react to milk products with back pain, neck pain, and headaches, and other symptoms. I know this to be unquestionably true. The exact mechanisms of the reaction, and what it is about milk that causes the reaction, are just theory, just my best guesses as I am attempting to explain. Just remember the premise, and consider that I may be wrong about the why's and wherefore's. I always consider that I may be wrong.

Getting back to margarine, look for possible reactions to whey. I haven't seen it a lot, but I have seen it. Some margarine manufacturers again cheat a little to make their product taste like what people are trying to avoid, that is, butter. One product, for example, called "I Can't Believe it's not Butter"™ is made with buttermilk. No wonder "I can't believe it's not butter." It is!

According to some experts, there are two kinds of allergy: fixed allergy and cyclic allergy. Once a person has developed a fixed allergy to a specific substance, any subsequent exposure will cause a reaction. For example, in a fixed allergy to penicillin, once a reaction has occurred, it will occur again, with no change in intensity, upon any exposure, no matter how much time has passed between exposures. In other words, the allergic response has not been diminished or eliminated by years of no exposure. A cyclic allergy is an allergic response that will disappear, or diminish after weeks, months, or years of no exposure. If a patient has an allergic headache of the cyclic variety, due to exposure to casein, abstinence from casein for a period of time, usually at least 3 to 4 months, will cause the allergy to disappear. This is an opinion shared by some allergists, not by me.

In his book, *How to Control Your Allergies,* Dr. Foreman describes fixed allergies as ones we are born with, ***not determined by previous exposure.*** Maybe some people are born with allergies, and maybe those allergies are the ones that are "fixed," and will always elicit a reaction. But I have seen sensitivities in infants that were eliminated when the offending foods were eliminated from the diet of the nursing mother. We know that casein, the milk protein, passes from mom's digestive tract into her breast milk and on to the nursing infant. Any food ingested by the mother, in fact, becomes part of the breast milk. I knew a woman who would drink a beer before nursing her baby, to induce sleep. Many infants who suffer from gas, diarrhea, colitis, or excema, and who cry a lot, and are obviously suffering, can get relief by eliminating casein from the diet of the nursing mother.

I think people who are born with allergies acquired them from exposure to the proteins that passed through the placenta into the system of the fetus, where the repeated exposure set off the allergy. We all know the terribly sad stories of infants who are born to drug users and are born addicted to drugs. These drugs have passed through the placenta from the drug-using mom to the fetus. So, although the baby was born with the addiction, the addiction was indeed caused by repeated previous exposure.

Many people tell me they "used to be allergic" to something. They know that, as a child, they had skin or digestive problems due to milk. But now, milk no longer causes problems for them. Sometimes, patients and doctors never find the culprit in infant food allergy, and even though the child continues to be exposed to the aggravating agent, the symptoms mysteriously disappear. Dr. Theron Randolph, the first one to extensively study food allergy, describes this phenomenon as "masking." He theorized that the allergic reaction has gone underground for several years to surface later as other symptoms. This is an interesting attempt to explain the weird nature of allergy.

Dr. Randolph's thinking illustrates how we in bio ecology think. We have seen the beast, and we know a few things about how it acts. Any theories we come up with are just attempts to explain the mechanisms of the phenomenon.

I tell patients that once you are allergic to something, you are always allergic to it. Some doctors believe that allergy is a childhood disease and is rare in adults because the allergy has been "outgrown." This is another attempt to explain the apparent disappearance of childhood allergy symptoms. We know that children who have problems with cow's milk in infancy (presumably allergy) can continue to drink it, but the symptoms seem to go away around the age of 5 or 6. These kids can continue to drink milk with "no apparent" problems. Many of these patients consult me in adolescence, or adulthood, with headaches, or back pain, that is, in fact, due to milk allergy.

The question, open to speculation and all these theories, is: "What happened in between infant sensitivity (colic, diarrhea, skin rashes) and adult sensitivity (headaches, back pain)?" It seems the symptoms went away then resurfaced. The first, and most difficult job, is to convince the patient that this is what actually happened. Don't even try to convince most medical doctors.

I think the symptoms didn't actually disappear between visits to the pediatrician, then to the chiropractor. In the developing infant, the digestive system seems to be the most susceptible, or at least the most *apparently* susceptible, to food allergies. If the allergen is affecting the nervous system, or the musculoskeletal system of an infant, how would you know? An infant is so uncoordinated anyway, as he or she is just experimenting with the new equipment. Arms and legs are flying everywhere. Watching a newborn is better than TV. Abnormalities would be difficult to spot. The infant can't speak to tell you about any pain or discomfort he or she is experiencing. And how would they know what's normal anyway? All they can do is squirm and cry, and these signals are important. Many parents assume that squirming and crying are normal baby activities, and sometimes they are. But again, how would a brand new parent know? We don't teach parenting in our schools.

Obviously.

A skin reaction, like excema, is obvious even to new parents, without any communication from the baby. So is diarrhea and gas. So these become the symptoms of infant allergy to milk because they are *apparent*. For some reason, as the digestive system develops, the sensitivity and symptoms decrease, or go away. The classic symptoms of the milk allergy begin manifesting themselves again, or anew, or they resurface, as chronic recurring ear infections, tonsilitis, asthma, and bronchitis in toddlers and 4 and 5 year olds. Conventional pediatricians hold to the thought of children outgrowing allergies. And, although some of these same doctors considered allergy as the culprit in infancy, they discount it in these toddlers. These conventional pediatricians prescribe medication, inhalers, instruct parents to use humidifiers, or dehumidifiers, they remove vital organs, like tonsils and appendices, and they insert tubes in these poor little guys' ears to drain the fluids of apparent infections. Once the tissues that have been inflamed are removed, the child is "cured."

Dr. J. Dan Baggett is a pediatrician in Alabama, and he has seen the milk connection. He says, "When I opened my practice here in Montgomery, Alabama, in 1960, I was aware of a causal relationship between cow-milk protein in the diet and infantile eczema. I also knew that many of these eczematoid children became asthmatics later on unless their eczema could be cleared early by dietary manipulation. This prompted me to begin a system of dietary prophylaxis against allergic disease among the newborns in my care.

"Only strained foods containing no milk, wheat, egg, or citrus were allowed through age nine months.

"When my babies developed eczema, they were promptly switched to a soy formula and although most of these did well, a few of them would clear, only to eventually develop eczema from the soy. Usually, there were further alternatives available, allowing me to raise them without eczema.

"Gradually, I became aware of the demonstrable relationship of food items in the causation of several respiratory and gastrointestinal disorders.

"In 1964, I learned of the experiences of Dr. William Deamer of San Francisco. He had pointed out the frequency of milk protein's causal relationship to musculoskeletal pain in children and especially the so called 'growing pains.'

"Since that time, I have had several children with what appeared to be early rheumatoid arthritis relieved and returned to good health by little more than reassurance and careful dietary manipulation.

"About six years ago, I began systematically persuading every patient of mine to delete all cow products from their diets. In general, they cooperate much better than I had earlier anticipated except for the preteenagers and teenagers.

"My patients are all given a list of 'legal' breads, crackers, cake mixes, cookies containing no casein, caseinate, whey, or milk solids. They are allowed small amounts of butter (contains 2 percent whey) and a 100 percent corn-oil margarine. Corn oil and safflower oil are recommended for cooking. They are, in addition, given a modification of Dr. W.L. Deamer's milk protein avoidance list to assist them in their shopping habits.

"During the years 1963 through 1967, I referred an average of four appendectomy cases per year. During the past five and a half years, I have referred only two patients for appendectomy, the last one being three years ago. Both of these children were professed milk guzzlers.

"I do not have a single patient with active asthma. In fact, I have nearly forgotten how to prescribe for them.

The Milk Connection

"Perhaps the most significant thing I have learned is that Group A beta-hemolytic streptococcus germ will not, under ordinary circumstances, establish an infection in a child kept on an absolutely no-milk-protein dietary regimen. I have been aware of this for the past two and a half years and, so far, there have been no exceptions. Any time a patient of mine is found to have streptococcal pharyngitis or pyoderma, we can establish by history that he has ingested milk protein within five days prior to the onset of symptoms or signs bringing him to the office.

"I now admit an average of 12-14 patients per year to the hospital. Their average hospital stay is three days. Between 1963 and 1967, I admitted an average of 100+ patients to the hospital per year. Their average hospital stay is five days.

"Breast fed is best fed and cow milk is the ideal food for the newly born and rapidly growing calf.

"My nursing mothers are advised to eat eggs, if tolerated, and dark green leafy vegetables and take prenatal vitamins and bone-meal tablets for an abundance of calcium. They are advised to eschew all cow-milk protein, chocolate, cola drinks, peanuts, and raw onion, and to eat anything else they want that doesn't upset their nursing baby. Such a wonderful experience is in store for them when they do it 'right.'

"The observation relating streptococcal disease to milk protein in the diet can be verified by most any pediatrician with time and patience to test it. It is often helpful to ask the child first whether he has had milk, ice cream, or cheese in his diet within the week prior to the office visit where strep is suspected. This cuts down on the embarrassment of having the child volunteer information contrary to the parent's story."[1]

The real "masking" years are the ages from about 7 to 14, the "wonder years." These kids seem to eat everything with "no apparent" problems. It's normal for a kid to be hyperactive, isn't it? Or to fall asleep in class, or to have a short attention

---

[1] Frank Oski, *Don't Drink Your Milk*, Mollica Press, Syracuse, N.Y. 1983

span, or need glasses, or have trouble hearing, or have trouble getting along with other kids, or to be seeing a therapist for dyslexia? Kids in this age range don't get much of an audience with adults. Their complaints, if they air them, or even recognize them as problems, especially minor ones, are usually signed off as kid stuff.

I believe that an infant, who demonstrates milk allergy with digestive and skin reactions, continues to suffer from the allergy in the wonder years with mucous disorders, ear infections, tonsilitis, appendicitis, etc. Some kids have chronic bad breath, no matter how often they brush their teeth. This is a classic symptom of milk allergy. I also believe that, if the child is allergic to casein, the allergy now has its affect on the rapidly developing nervous system, causing symptoms like learning and behavior disorders. Many times, in fact most times, these symptoms are not so severe that the child is jailed, just enough to cause him or her or their parents or teachers some inconvenience, perhaps.

A 5 or 6 year old with glasses? Not normal. To me, probably the "not so apparent" reaction to the allergen that is affecting the lens, or the fluid in the eyeball, or the blood vessels of the retina. Most people can accept certain symptoms as possible allergy, like hives and runny noses, and still others can be talked into considering headaches. But to suggest that other "not so apparent" symptoms, like learning disorders, behavior problems, and poor vision, doesn't fit comfortably into most peoples' belief systems. I think the kids in the wonder years, who seem to be unaffected by allergy, suffer the most. Many of them experience growing pains, and we tell them that's normal. But I have treated many kids with back pain and joint pain, 13 year olds that move like old men, they get bloody noses. These are more classic symptoms of allergy to milk in adolescence, totally relieved by abstinence from all dairy products. Sadly enough, many of them are forced to eat the foods that are causing them problems, mainly milk. Most school lunch programs offer only one choice of drinks for lunch — milk.

At puberty, the hormone changes kick in, causing those awkward changes that transform kids into adults, the metamorphosis that produces that amazing phenomenon, the teenager. Boys are holding hands with girls who stand a head taller than them. What is normal behavior at a junior high school is anybody's guess. I was a pretty good kid, but I think I confused my parents and some of my teachers while I was at Fort Miller Junior High. Dermatologists have made a great living treating teenagers and their skin problems, mainly acne, that seem to occur when the hormones are dumped into the system. Most of the kids are scrubbing, using ointments, jells, infra red lights, etc. Parents are lining the pockets of dermatologists for about 4 years when, all of a sudden, the skin miraculously clears. Amazingly, some dermatologists actually consider the diet. But the changes they recommend reflect that they don't really consider dietary causes as allergy. They usually recommend cutting out chocolate, sweets, and cutting back on milk, seldom mentioning cheese and yogurt and other casein containing foods, and seldom following up with continuing dietary analysis.

After the skin clears, as it does in most people (some aren't so lucky) the allergy continues and becomes apparent, at least to me, as musculoskeletal pain, or headaches, usually. Patients I see complain of headaches, neck and back pain, arthritic joints, arm and/or leg numbness, etc. I'm sure there are many other symptoms of the allergy that go unnoticed, or that are showing up in other doctors' offices.

The allergy manifests itself in middle aged patients as continuing, and now chronic, joint and back pain, heart disorders, varicose veins, endometriosis, and decreased energy. There seems to be a strong link between allergy and the female hormone system. Many women, and their families, suffer from premenstrual syndrome (PMS) during their monthly cycle, usually about a week before the menstrual flow. During this time, sufferers act inappropriately, they are quick to anger, they suffer from cramps. Many of these women experience intense cravings during this time, many times for chocolate, or salty foods, or sweets. In taking histories over the years, I have seen a high incidence of endometriosis, varicose veins, and ovarian cysts, and skin cysts, in women who suffer from musculoskeletal pain due to allergy to casein. I'm not the only one who has seen this. Dr. Christiane Northrup, M.D., an obstetrician and gynecologist from Portland says, "Dairy products seem very much associated with menstrual cramps and heavy flow." Also, breast tenderness and swelling has been alleviated when dairy products were eliminated from the diet.

Annemarie Colbin, a nutritionist, says, "Even fertility appears to have been reversed with this approach in several instances — not so strange when you consider that in some cases infertility results from the fallopian tubes being blocked by mucus. When the mucus caused by dairy foods clears up, conception is more likely to occur. In addition to its macronutrients, milk, being a product of the reproductive glands, also contains an appreciable amount of hormones, including gonadotropins, thyroid releasing hormones, ovarian steroids, and an epidermal growth factor. What role the growth factor may have in the development of gross overweight or cancer has not yet been investigated, but I suspect we may be hearing more on the subject in the future."

I treated a patient recently for headaches. Pam had been married for nine years, trying to get pregnant the entire time. The closest she came was two miscarriages. Seven months prior to consulting me, she had read *Fit for Life,* an excellent diet book written by Harvey and Marilyn Diamond. The Diamonds write that "cow's milk is unfit for human consumption." After changing her diet, Pam conceived, and was five months along when she first consulted me. Her headaches went beyond the milk connection, but she did get total relief from her headaches with dietary manipulation. Her case appears in the story section.

Many 40 and 50 year old women I treat, who suffer with musculoskeletal pain due to milk allergy, are taking thyroid hormones. Some have been diagnosed as suffering from Epstein-Barr virus, or chronic fatigue syndrome. These two diagnoses, and thyroid deficiencies, are becoming more and more popular. But the symptoms, diagnostic tests, and treatment programs are so vague that I can't, for the life of me, figure out why these diagnoses seem more plausible to the medical profession than allergy. There is no question in my mind that most, if not all, of these disorders are manifestations of allergy.

In this same age group, and older, many people suffer with neurological symptoms that occur so often that they have been named. Medical textbooks are full of these disorders with fancy names, like Guillain Barré syndrome, Meniere's syndrome, Raynaud's phenomenon, multiple sclerosis, and many, many more. All these neurological disorders have one thing in common: cause unknown. When you get to the symptom chapter (Chapter 4) in this book, you will see some of these disorders without their name tags: ringing in the ears (medics call this Meniere's), tingling and numbness in the hands and/or feet (Guillain Barré or Raynaud's), decreased energy level (thyroid dysfunction, or Epstein-Barr).

Many older Americans suffer with Parkinson's Disease, or Alzheimer's: cause, deterioration of parts of the brain. Cause of deterioration of the brain? Unknown. Alcohol can do it. Trauma can do it. I recently read an article about one of the greatest, most influential men of all time, Muhammad Ali. The fact that he was merely a boxer does not, in my mind, detract from the qualities that make him great. The boxing ring served only as an arena to put him in the spot light, so we could enjoy his greatness and learn from him. At this writing, he suffers from Parkinson's disease. In this disease, the normally finely tuned fluid movements (of which he was the master) have become jerky and uncontrollable. These sufferers are unable to hold their heads still, their hands shake. Ali suffers with it, but doesn't complain. He offers no excuses for this, or any of his defeats. He just accepts, and moves on. The article mentions briefly that Ali partakes each and every day of his favorite snack, apple pie a la mode.

I just observe.

No Milk

I really don't feel I have had enough experience to make an accurate conclusion about some of these disorders, I treat musculoskeletal disorders, but I can tell you what I have seen and what I think. First of all, if a patient sees me for, lets say, low back pain, and we establish that the pain is an allergic reaction to casein, the patient gets better through treatment and abstinence from dairy products and is released. Several things can happen after a patient is released.

1) Most often these patients return at some later date when they have returned to using dairy products in their diets and the same symptoms have recurred. Amazingly enough, the time between release and return is three months, not always, but very often. Again, the treatment is the same, adjustments and instructions to completely abstain from dairy products. These patients are now usually convinced that the milk connection is real, and will make a concerted effort to stay away from milk products. As a result, they will not experience their "chronic" problem.

Many patients need the proof of a reaction after re-exposure to dairy products to become convinced that the milk connection is real. After they have successfully avoided dairy products, received chiropractic treatment, then get better, they wonder if changing their diets really had anything to do with their symptoms.

It reminds me of a scene from *Dirty Harry,* when Clint Eastwood shoots it out with a bad guy. After all the excitement, he has his gun trained on the bad guy, but can't remember if he used all his bullets, or has one left in the chamber of his .44 Magnum. The bad guy surrenders, but as Dirty Harry is about to walk away, the bad guy's curiosity overwhelms him. He says, "I just gots to know."

After they get better, some patients just "gots to know," so they walk into the Häagen Dazs™ store and pull the trigger. Then they know.

It is very common for patients to return in three months or so after they were released. Their symptoms have returned, and they don't know why. Dietary questioning reveals that they have returned to using dairy products, causing their symptoms to return. Somehow, they seemed to have forgotten the milk connection.

2) Some patients will follow my dietary suggestions for a short period of time, until they recover, then are released. They will return several years later with similar symptoms and report that they have been using dairy products since their release, but not as much, and they've been okay until some physical trauma set off their pain again. Same treatment: adjustments, no dairy. They get better.

3) The patients that get better, then return to using dairy with no further problems, seldom contact me. Maybe that happens, I just don't know. But sometimes, after a patient recovers and is released, we get a slip in the mail from another doctor requesting our records. I have had the opportunity to speak with some of these patients. Most of them don't really want to talk to me. They just think I'm crazy. "Well, I tried your diet and it didn't work." I'm sure that happens sometimes, this isn't a cure-all. But when patients let me manage their cases and their diets for a reasonable period of time, I see failure to comply over 70% of the time.

Many patients slip, "Oops, didn't know there was cheese on that sandwich until I ate the whole thing." Others give in to temptation. It is the rare patient who is 100% successful in their first attempt to totally abstain from dairy foods.

Many patients just "cut back" for a period of time, don't get better, then totally discount the notion that their pain is related to their diets. They seem to think, despite my explanation, that if they cut back, they will see a commensurate decrease in symptoms. "Told you so. I didn't think it made any sense at all." They feel they proved me wrong, which many times, oddly enough, seems to be their goal. Weird, huh?

I saw one patient who suffered from low back pain after an auto accident. Although she really thought I was out of my mind, I got her to stay off dairy products for a month. She recovered and was released after I was able to point out several reactions of low back pain that she experienced after exposure to dairy foods. Four months after her release, she came in to get her records because she was consulting another chiropractor for the same injury. I was baffled. She had gone back to using dairy products shortly after I released her. When her pain returned, she didn't want to hear my story. When she consulted the next chiropractor, she told him what I had told her about dairy products. She said he was shocked. He told her she would suffer more if she didn't drink her milk to prevent osteoporosis. Of course, in her eyes, I was wrong and he was right. I told her that it was my opinion that if she continued to drink milk, she would continue to have pain. That completely destroyed my credibility with her, and the chiropractic community here has some doubts about my work.

And I thought they would steal my discovery! Silly me.

Another patient came to see me complaining of severe shoulder and neck pain. He had seen chiropractors before for the same problem and knew it just needed to be "snapped back in place." I adjusted him and instructed him to eliminate dairy products from his diet for at least 30 days. He returned in 22 days and said, "Well, I tried your diet for a month, and I was real good, and it didn't help."

I looked at the dates on his chart. "So, you're back using dairy products again?", I asked.

"Yeah."

"How long have you been back on dairy products?"

"About two or three weeks."

Writing everything down is a good idea, because most of us have pretty poor memories and a poor sense of time. This patient evidently missed his dairy products and had suffered for, what seemed to him, to be weeks and weeks without them. Luckily, I write everything down and gave him the numbers that had to do with time. Looking at the dates, and his report, he may have avoided dairy products for one to two weeks — maybe. If he was one of the rare people who successfully avoids **ALL** casein without guidance, he just may have given the milk connection a sufficient test, but probably not.

When I explained the rules of the game to him, he gave it a better shot. And guess what? He's no longer a patient, except that time he came in last Easter after eating a chocolate bunny. Expensive bunny.

So what are the rules of the milk connection? If the symptoms that a patient is experiencing are due, in part, or completely, to an allergic reaction to casein, how much time must pass before these symptoms change? The time of recovery is important to a patient. It is very difficult to get a patient to give up a food he or she loves. Milk seems to be one of those foods that most users not only love, but lust after. I have had many, many patients look at me and sigh, "No way. I can't live without my milk."

Maybe that's true, and sometimes a patient will flat out **refuse** to give up milk. But most of them can be convinced to give up dairy products for a short period of time, if they know they can eventually go back to them. It's my job to see if I can convince them that the milk connection is real, and that the benefit to them will be worth the sacrifice. That is a big job.

This is the story I tell: "I didn't make this up. In fact, when I first heard Mr. Ester tell me his pain was caused by milk, I didn't believe him. The fact is, I have seen over 3000 different people who experienced neck pain, back pain, joint pain, and/or headaches due to milk. When these patients eliminated dairy products from their diets, 95% of them experienced a complete remission from their complaints."

This is not a statement I make to all patients regardless of their complaints. I make this statement to patients who I have interviewed thoroughly, then determined that there is a connection between their symptoms and their diets. The patient needs to know the following information about the milk connection:

1) **reaction time,**
2) **foods that will cause the reaction,**
3) **duration of the reaction, and**
4) **recovery time after milk is eliminated**

First, we must establish the cause of the symptoms, whether it is a traumatic event, or a dietary event. This is sometimes difficult to do. Most patients assume that physical symptoms are due to physical trauma, and most of them have a story to tell me about what they feel caused their symptoms. They have already picked out a traumatic event that preceded and seemed to cause their complaints. I go over this trauma with the patient to establish the causal relationship between it and their complaints. Most times there is a definite relationship.

Many times this relationship is obvious, like a patient who never suffered with neck pain and headaches until one hour after the car he or she was driving was rear ended. Several years ago, I used to discount a dietary connection in these cases and proceed with conventional treatment using manipulation and physical therapy. But the normal response in all but the most severe whiplash should, in my opinion, be like the recovery from a sprained ankle. A sprained ankle is acutely sore and swollen for two to three weeks, then gradually gets better until a complete recovery has taken place in six months or less. But it was not a rare occurrence in my office to see patients who were still suffering with neck pain and headaches many years after a seemingly minor whip lash accident.

So now, despite the traumatic history of a patient, I **always** consider a dietary connection. To establish a dietary connection, I first must establish the occurrence and frequency of symptoms. When the symptoms come and go, I try to isolate a specific recurrence of the symptoms, then establish the diet around the time of the symptoms. Usually, a patient comes into the office because he or she is experiencing symptoms. We first establish when the symptoms began. I try to establish the date and the hour. If the patient can pin it down within the last three or four days, we have a very good chance of recovering a fairly accurate report of foods eaten in that time period from the patient's memory. When a patient has suffered with pain for a week or more, hoping it would go away, establishing the diet at the time of the onset is very difficult. Most people, including myself, don't remember what they ate two days ago, much less a week ago. But in relentless questioning, several tools will help the patient remember what they have eaten. I often ask if they ate out or at home, did they go to a friend's house, or to a party? I also consider holidays, like Easter, Christmas, Halloween, Thanksgiving, etc. It helps to have a friend or relative present to help remember what was happening around the time of onset of symptoms. When we establish a date and time, we analyze the diet before the onset of pain.

Reaction time. This is the time that passes between ingestion of a food and a patient's reaction to it. When a patient ingests a food to which he or she is sensitive, symptoms will occur anytime between instantaneously, to 48 hours. Typical reaction time is two to twelve hours. When the time of onset of symptoms is established, I attempt to establish what foods were eaten prior to the onset, beginning with the meal immediately prior to the pain. I then work backwards in time, attempting to accurately, and completely establish everything the patient ate.

By far, the most common story I hear is that the onset of pain was in the morning. The patients usually report that they woke up with pain, or couldn't get out of bed, or threw their backs out in the shower, or at the sink, or when they bent down to pick up the newspaper. The most common story is that the pain began before breakfast. I start with establishing what the patient ate for supper the night before. This is usually where the culprit was eaten, if indeed there is a dietary connection. There usually is. However, going back in time over the foods that were eaten will sometimes uncover the cases of slower onset. These cases are not as common as the typical two to twelve hour reaction time, but they do happen. The culprit could have been eaten as much as 48 hours before the reaction.

Foods that cause a reaction. As I have stated over and over again, the number one cause of neck pain, back pain and headaches is milk and dairy products. Of all the dairy products that cause symptoms, the number one most powerful, by far, 100 times more powerful than all the rest, is **chocolate.** I make this statement because the cases with the most sudden and most acute symptoms are usually preceded by the ingestion of chocolate. Based on that same criterion, number two is **ice cream,** and number three is **sour cream.**

The busiest day in my schedule is November 1, the day after Halloween. The busiest week in my schedule is the week after Easter Sunday. These holidays are celebrated with lots of chocolate. What is it about chocolate that makes it so powerful? Many doctors know that chocolate can cause headaches. But when their patients eliminate it, the response is usually not 100%. The best response is that the headaches are not as frequent and/or not as severe, but seldom does eliminating chocolate completely eliminate headaches. However, most doctors and patients consider any improvement a success.

What is in chocolate, anyway? The main ingredient in chocolate is cocoa, which contains a couple of powerful stimulants, caffeine and theobromine. Milk chocolate contains cocoa, cream, milk solids, and sugar. I know that patients who react to milk and dairy products also react to chocolate, only worse. So it seems that eliminating milk chocolate is indicated, and that other forms of chocolate will not cause a reaction in milk sensitive patients. Unfortunately, this is not true. It seems that all forms of chocolate cause severe reactions.

Is chocolate an allergen, or a poison? Are reactions to it allergy to casein, or cocoa, or are they reactions to the powerful stimulants, theobromine and caffeine? New wave allergists commonly use the term "allergy-addiction" because, many times, the foods we are allergic to, we are also addicted to. Many people know they are "chocoholics" and experience intense cravings for it. Chocolate not only causes neck pain, back pain, and headaches in sensitive people, but can also cause irritability, depression, and anxiety. Many "chocoholics" experience mood swings, becoming irritable and snapping at loved ones for no apparent reason. "I'm just crabby." Many women, for some reason, crave chocolate around their menstrual cycles. They then become irritable, depressed, and anxious, and are told they have PMS, premenstrual syndrome.

The word "syndrome" appears in many diagnoses. Syndrome is only a collection of symptoms and in no way implies that doctors know the cause. In fact, if you see the word "syndrome" in a diagnosis, you can be sure that the cause is unknown. The doctor has just managed to list your symptoms and give it a name. Premenstrual Syndrome is one of the most poorly understood conditions. I don't pretend to understand it any more than anyone else, but I know in many cases PMS is only a reaction to foods that are craved by the victim. Many, many, many times, that food is chocolate.

People who react to milk and dairy products with back pain, neck pain, and/or headaches, also react in the same way to chocolate, only worse. I have seen only two patients who claim they react to dairy products, but not to chocolate.

So, I just told you everything I know about chocolate. Is it a poison or an allergen? I don't know. I think reactions to chocolate are a combination of allergy and reactions to the powerful stimulants. I think this combined effect is what makes the reaction so severe in some people. I could be wrong. I can only make one solid conclusion about it:

Don't eat chocolate.

When I see a patient who is suffering excruciating pain, that came on all of a sudden for no apparent reason, it is almost always preceded by the ingestion of chocolate.

Although I said that allergic reactions are not dose dependent, it seems that some foods are more powerful than others. **Chocolate is number one, ice cream is number two, and sour cream is number three.** The most severe reactions occur after chocolate and ice cream are combined, a very common combination in this country. Vanilla ice cream with chocolate syrup, "Cookies 'n Cream™ ice cream," "Fudge Ripple™," neopolitan ice cream, or brownies and ice cream are snacks that commonly precede the onset of severe neck pain, back pain, joint pain, and/or headaches. It seems that when an allergen, like casein, is combined with sugar and/or a stimulant, the reaction is more powerful. It also seems that the reaction is more severe when the percentage of casein in the dairy food is higher. Solid dairy foods, like cheeses, have a higher concentration of casein because the liquid portion, the whey, has been eliminated, leaving a higher percentage of protein.

	%protein	%water
Parmesan cheese	36	30
Swiss cheese	27.5	39.9
Cheddar (American) cheese	25	37
Brick cheese	22.2	41
Blue or Roquefort cheese	21.5	40
Domestic Camembert cheese	17.5	52.2
Creamed Cottage cheese	13.6	78.3
Cream cheese	8.0	51
Canned Condensed Sweetened Milk	8.1	27.1
Canned Evaporated Unsweetened Milk	7.0	73.8
Skim Milk	3.6	90.5
Fluid Cultured Buttermilk	3.6	90.5
Whole Milk	3.5	87.4
Light Whipping Cream	2.5	62.1
Unsalted Butter	0.6	15.5

In spot checking meals, the entire meal must be accounted for:

"What did you have for dinner last night?"

"Chicken."

"Anything else?"

"Rice."

"Did you have a salad?"

"Yeah."

"Dressing?"

"Ranch?" (made with buttermilk)

It must be established what they drank, vegetables, desert, etc.

I always ask patients if they are on any kind of a special diet. Many times, after reporting that they don't use dairy products, they report that they are taking some kind of protein shake once or several times a day, mixed with milk.

Once, after grilling a patient about his diet and establishing that dairy products had been eliminated, I decided that I was not going to see a dietary connection to justify the severe recurrence of his back pain. This patient had been a big ice cream eater, and after I had finally convinced him to give it up, he also gave up his "chronic" back condition and about 17 pounds. But here he was again, one year later with the same symptoms and, as he reported, no use of dairy products. After I gave up questioning him, using every technique I knew, I kept talking about food and pain, explaining that chocolate was the most powerful cause of the severe pain that he was experiencing.

"Well," he said, "the only chocolate I use is in this protein shake I have been taking for two weeks now."

"You've been eating chocolate?" I was aghast. "What do you mix it with?"

"Low fat milk."

"How often do you have this protein drink?"

"Just twice a day."

So after eliminating dairy products successfully for a year, he was now having milk and chocolate every day, again. But, I guess since it wasn't a candy bar, or cake, or ice cream he didn't consider that he was eating chocolate and milk. I guess. I sometimes wonder how many of these patients walk out the door with neither of us discovering the truth.

No Milk

I have seen many patients who began experiencing low back pain one or several weeks after starting a diet program of Slim Fast™, or Ultra Slim Fast™. These protein shakes are mixed with milk. The powdered portion itself contains sodium caseinate. Most people choose chocolate flavor. So with an increase in milk intake, usually twice a day, and a double daily dose of chocolate, the most powerful dairy food, it takes only a few days or weeks to react.

It is very helpful when a relative accompanies the patient and can remember things the patient can't, or is willing to "tell on" the patient. Wives and husbands are usually great tattlers. I once treated a 43 year old man for a recurring low back problem that radiated as pain and numbness into his right leg. We eliminated dairy products from his diet and treated him for three weeks. He completely recovered and was released. Six months later he returned on a Friday, reporting that he was experiencing some right leg discomfort for about a week. After intense questioning to establish a dietary connection, he persisted in claiming that he was not using dairy products. I adjusted his back and instructed him to return on Monday for treatment. On Monday he returned in severe pain. He was in such severe pain that he could not drive. His son had driven him in. The patient reported to me that on Saturday, following treatment, he felt much better. He went to bed on Saturday night feeling good. He woke up Sunday morning in severe pain. Now, on Monday, he was still in severe pain. So here we have an isolated exacerbation in recent memory. The questions began.

"What did you have for dinner on Saturday night?"

"We went out for dinner. I had prime rib."

"Baked potato?" My thinking here, is that severe pain was probably caused by one of the top three, chocolate, ice cream, or sour cream. Baked potatoes are often dressed with sour cream.

"Yeah, I had a baked potato with salt and pepper, no butter, no sour cream." (He had been through this before with me.)

"Did you have a salad?"

"Yeah."

"Dressing?"

"Oil and vinegar."

Still nothing.

"Any dessert?"

"No. nothing."

His son, sitting quietly until now, became the rat. "Yes you did, Dad."

"I did? What did I have?"

"Bavarian cream pie."

"That makes more sense," I responded, relieved. "You had chocolate, whipped cream, and evaporated milk in that pie. Now I understand why you woke up with severe pain on Sunday. I still don't understand why you had pain last week, though, since you had no dairy and no chocolate."

The rat came back, "Yes you did, Dad. Remember last week you ate that whole bag of Hershey's Kisses™?"

Oh, good, I'm not crazy after all.

I learn more things every day about taking a more accurate history. Later I will list questions I commonly use to establish dietary habits and attain other useful information. Many times a patient will suddenly remember a food he or she ate, but had neglected during the initial questioning. Many, many times, I will be explaining how chocolate is the most powerful agent, and the patient will suddenly respond, "You know, I *did* have some chocolate."

The aggravating agent in cow's milk is casein. Casein is used as an additive in many foods to give them added flavor, the flavor found in cow's milk. The additive will be listed on the label, usually as sodium caseinate, or calcium caseinate. Many times the manufacturer will actually put in parentheses after sodium caseinate "(a milk derivative)". All powdered non-dairy creamers use sodium caseinate, or potassium caseinate, or calcium caseinate to give them the taste and consistency of milk. Many liquid coffee creamers also use the milk derivative.

Diet mayonnaise and many packaged foods use this additive that will cause a reaction in a person sensitive to casein.

So a doctor's advice to "cut back" on milk products is usually insufficient advice. Many times doctors believe that aged cheeses and chocolates can cause headaches. What these foods have in common is the milk protein, casein, and unless all casein is eliminated, the results will be poor.

Duration of Reaction. Like reaction time, and sensitivity, the duration of the reaction will vary in different people. When a person is sensitive to a food allergen, a single exposure typically causes symptoms that begin in 2 to 12 hours, and persist for 3 to 4 days. When a food is ingested, it takes about four days to be digested, absorbed, then reabsorbed from the tissue and excreted. It may cause a reaction and symptoms during its entire stay in the body. Because of this, it should be understood that symptoms can become constant, then diagnosed as chronic, when a patient eats dairy products only two or three times a week! Most doctors and patients consider this frequency to be very light, and therefor insufficient to be considered a cause of a chronic complaint.

Some people, who are less sensitive, may have symptoms that will come and go in a few hours. Most people who react to casein with a headache, will suffer with it for one day. The following day, the headache will be decreased, or gone. This is assuming, of course, that the patient doesn't renew the reaction by continuing to eat foods with casein.

Recovery time after milk is eliminated. The only way to eliminate symptoms that are due to a reaction to casein is, of course, to totally eliminate all casein from the diet. This doesn't mean cut back. It means totally eliminate. This means eliminate all milk, including on cereal and in coffee, all non-dairy creamers that use sodium caseinate, cheese, cottage cheese, cream cheese, sour cream, ranch dressing, bleu cheese, ice cream, ice milk, sherbet, yogurt, frozen yogurt, butter, buttermilk, chocolate, caramel, pizza, and on and on, all of it, every single drop. Breads that contain milk, and many do, must be eliminated.

Most donuts are made with milk. Biscuits, gravy, mashed potatoes, pancakes, etc. All the good stuff. Fattening, tasty.

You know, it couldn't be liver or spinach.

Once a person who is sensitive to casein has successfully, totally eliminated casein from his or her diet (no small task, by the way), symptoms due to that sensitivity will disappear in 7 to 30 days.

So, what happens in the first seven days?

Withdrawal.

Withdrawal?

You got to be kidding!

Withdrawal. When a person is sensitive to a particular substance, he or she will experience withdrawal symptoms when that substance is eliminated. This is a phenomenon of allergy-addiction.

Most of us have heard of the intense withdrawal a heroin addict goes through when he or she quits the drug, or can't get it. A typical heroin addict gets a fix every day. When he or she doesn't get the fix on time, withdrawal begins. The addict breaks out in a cold sweat, gets the shivers, feels terrible, and has an intense craving for heroin. The addict will do just about anything during this withdrawal to get a fix. Why? Because a fix will end the miserable withdrawal symptoms. This fix is the "neutralizing dose." So the addict has two choices, it seems: To experience the "high" or nirvana, the symptoms of the drug when under the influence of heroin, or to suffer the misery of withdrawal when the drug is not available. The third choice of the heroin addict, of course, is to quit "cold turkey." To do this, the addict must ride out the withdrawal. If he or she makes it to the other side, to sobriety, the roller coaster ride of addiction-withdrawal is over. Over, that is, as long as heroin is completely avoided.

Many of the new wave allergists, the bio-ecologists, believe that alcoholism is a classic example of allergy-addiction. The typical alcoholic drinks every day to get drunk, or high, or to satisfy his or her "need." After they pass out, or sleep it off, they wake up and experience that wonderful feeling called "hangover." This is the beginning of withdrawal, a condition I describe as "an overall feeling of lousiness." If the severely addicted alcoholic remains dry, the symptoms worsen over the next few days. Withdrawal for the severe alcoholic may involve delirium tremens (the DT's), severe shakes, hallucinations, severe headaches, and, of course, an intense craving for alcohol. When the alcoholic awakes with a hangover, he or she can end this "overall feeling of lousiness" by having a shot of booze, or a beer, an "eye opener." I think this is how Bloody Mary's became popular as a breakfast drink. This morning drink becomes the neutralizing dose, and withdrawal, the hangover, is temporarily staved off.

In the theory of alcoholism as allergy-addiction, we believe the aggravating agent, or the allergen, is the particular grain of the alcoholic beverage. Most alcoholics have their favorite drink, whether it's beer, or whisky, or whatever. The alcoholic is suffering from allergy to the particular grain of their favorite drink. Once exposure to that grain is stopped, the roller coaster ride of allergy-addiction, drunk-hangover, symptom-withdrawal, will stop, and sobriety will be the reward. However, if the alcoholic continues to expose him or her self to the aggravating grain in other foods, like breads, the craving will continue. In this case, only a strong willed person will be able to remain dry.

The phenomenon of allergy-addiction involves these highs and lows no matter what the substance. Many people are aware of, or have experienced the withdrawal from caffeine when they quit drinking coffee. Most regular coffee drinkers are aware of the craving they have for it. Many people feel they just can't get started in the morning without their "fix", their cup of coffee. I've had people tell me that they tried to do without coffee for a few days, and just couldn't survive. They had no energy, they felt lousy, they had a headache, They interpret this to mean that their bodies "need" coffee.

Well, the coffee drinker's body doesn't need coffee any more than the heroin addict's body needs heroin. The feeling of "need", or craving, happens because of withdrawal. People who have successfully quit caffeine after years of use, probably experienced the withdrawal headache. This headache usually lasts for three to four days, sometimes as long as seven days. So when a person says they cannot make it without coffee, or their body needs it, or they feel worse without it, they are describing the withdrawal effects of allergy-addiction to caffeine. They will do just fine without it, probably better than ever, if they can make it through seven days of withdrawal.

Withdrawal from milk and dairy products is similar to withdrawal from caffeine. Classic withdrawal is a headache on the third day of abstinence from all casein in dairy products. This third day withdrawal headache is usually pretty severe. Typically, it lasts all day on the third day, then is diminished or gone on the fourth day. But some people experience a headache for seven days, or on the fifth and sixth day of withdrawal. Other people don't get a headache. Some people experience an overall feeling of lousiness, like a hangover, or like they're coming down with a cold or the flu. Some people actually get cold symptoms. I have had many patients cancel an appointment on the 3rd or 4th day of withdrawal because they have a cold. Some people experience severe back pain in withdrawal, although this is rare.

The withdrawal symptoms can occur any time during the first seven days. Some patients have reported that they experienced withdrawal for more than seven days, but this is rare. It's possible that these people re-exposed themselves to casein during withdrawal without knowing it. I once saw a 50 year old man who had suffered with severe back pain for 10 years. He was a recovering alcoholic. He smoked three packs of cigarettes a day, and ate five or six chocolate candy bars every day. He drank a gallon of milk a day. Believe it or not, I was able to convince him to eliminate dairy products and choc- olate from his diet. He reported severe withdrawal symptoms for three weeks. This could have been because he was with- drawing from the most powerful dairy food, chocolate. Maybe part of his withdrawal had to do with withdrawal from theobromine, the powerful and poorly understood stimulant in chocolate. Maybe it had to do with his other addictions. Maybe it had to do with the fact that he had heavily exposed himself to chocolate and dairy products for years. I don't know, but I have only seen this three week withdrawal once, but must consider that it could happen.

This patient recovered from his back pain in five weeks. It was a tough, long haul. I had never seen such a slow response, and, quite frankly, I was worried during the whole process. Several years later, his daughter was seeing me as a patient. She informed me that he had suffered three heart attacks in a three month period. The damage had been done.

So, to put all of this in a nutshell, I tell patients the following:

1) All casein, in all forms, must be totally eliminated.

2) Withdrawal will take place for 7 days. (Possibly longer)

3) Symptoms that are due to allergy to casein will disappear in seven to thirty days. If symptoms do not change in 30 days, they will not change by eliminating casein.

"So, what if I do all this and I don't get better?"

This is a common question, and a good one. A successful case depends not only on good treatment, but, more importantly, good management. I manage these cases by first taking a thorough history, as I have explained. A thorough history is the most powerful diagnostic tool in medicine — bar none. Better than x-ray, blood tests, MRI, all that high tech stuff. A good history will determine the cause of disease. If the doctor doesn't know the cause, she can't eliminate it. The most common medical case proceeds right into treatment with the cause unknown. Typical medical treatment only treats symptoms and completely glosses over the cause.

This same mentality would seem ludicrous in real life. Imagine, an M.D. was driving down the road when all of a sudden his oil indicator light came on. After several miles, the light was still on. The doctor rapped on the instrument panel trying to get the light to shut off. Finally, he realized he was going to have to get at the cause of the problem, so he pulled over to the side of the road and opened his trunk. He selected a Phillips head screwdriver to perform the operation. He proceeded to the cockpit where he disassembled the instrument panel and removed the troublesome light bulb. He replaced the dashboard cover, put the tools away, slammed the trunk shut, and proceeded to the golf course with a satisfied air. "Gee, I didn't know I was a great mechanic, too!"

Of course, he did not address the real cause of the problem by changing or adding oil, he just eliminated the indicator, the symptom. Many medical cases are treated in this manner.

When I believe that casein is the cause of a patient's complaints, I instruct the patient, as above, to avoid casein and expect withdrawal and all that we've discussed. I tell them the whole story. I take note of the date of their last use of dairy foods, and enter on their charts the date of Day 1, the first day of abstinence.

I have them return in several days, depending on their symptoms, anywhere from one to seven days after the first visit. If the second visit takes place more than seven days after the first visit, the patient's memory will be vague, and so will the case. On the second visit I basically take another history about what has transpired in the days since the first visit. I ask them to describe the ebb and flow of their symptoms. I ask them what they ate. I ask more detailed questions to clarify what they ate.

I'm looking for several things, first, possible exposure to casein. About 70% of the time, despite the patient's best attempts, the diet has been violated. I look for this violation to point out a possible reaction to the casein, to show the milk connection, and to show how difficult it is to avoid all casein. If the patient has "slipped", I think it's important to point out the source of their exposure to help them be more successful in their attempt. The violation will usually be some innocuous form of casein, like mashed potatoes made with milk.

No Milk

Sometimes, though, a seemingly obvious violation has occurred without the patient's knowledge.

I once treated a 47 year old man who complained of low back pain that radiated into his right leg. I saw him first on a Monday. After taking a thorough history, I treated him and instructed him to avoid all milk and dairy products. He returned two days later on Wednesday for his second treatment. He reported at that time that he had some low back discomfort, but that the leg pain was gone. After questioning him about the foods he had been eating, I was satisfied that he was successfully avoiding all casein. He returned two days later, on Friday, and showed more improvement and was still avoiding dairy products. He was to return the following Monday, but cancelled due to his work schedule. He came in two days later on Wednesday. I asked him how he was. "Good today," he said. "But I woke up on Monday morning with back and leg pain, just like before. And I didn't do anything physical to cause it."

"What did you have for supper on Sunday night?" I asked.

"I don't remember."

"Well, think about it, and I'll be back."

When I returned in five minutes, I asked him again, "Did you remember what you had on Sunday night?"

"Pizza." He said it with the blankest expression I have ever seen.

"I rest my case," I responded.

"What do you mean?"

"Remember I told you to avoid all dairy products because I thought your pain was caused by casein?"

"Yeah. What? Is there milk in the crust of pizza or something?" He looked puzzled.

"No. There's cheese all over the top of it."

"Oh yeah!" He was surprised. "Actually" he went on, "I really didn't believe that stuff about dairy products, but I was doing it anyway. Wow, I can't believe it. Do you really think that's it?"

It seems obvious that pizza is loaded with dairy products, but I have seen many people miss it. I understand it, though. For two years, I gave patients a typed list of dairy products to avoid. I made no mention of pizza!

When asking people about their weekly use of cheese, some respond that they use it "maybe once a week." Then I'll say just one word, "Pizza?"

"Oh yeah, pizza."

The questioning on the second visit is also designed to uncover other possible causes of the patient's complaints. Casein is the number one cause of back pain, neck pain, and headaches. In my experience, casein causes these symptoms in 95% of cases. But it cannot be assumed that the patient is not one of the other 5%. Believe it or not, the other 5% of these cases are caused, usually, by other dietary poisons, or allergens. When a particular exacerbation of pain occurs between the first and second visits, thorough questioning must be used to isolate the cause, whether it was a physical event, withdrawal, or exposure to casein, or exposure to another poison or allergen.

When a patient experiences an exacerbation three or four or five days after the first visit, the cause is most likely withdrawal, especially if the exacerbation is a symptom other than the original complaint. For example, a patient who originally complains of chronic low back pain on the first visit, then experiences a severe headache on the third day, has probably experienced withdrawal from casein. This, however, cannot be assumed. Withdrawal doesn't happen in every case. Some patients show immediate improvement after one treatment and as soon as dairy products are eliminated from the diet. A headache three or four days later could be due to re-exposure to casein. This must be determined by a thorough questioning of the diet, especially the meal prior to the onset of the headache.

Edna, a 54 year old female came in to consult me about her chronic low back pain. She had consulted her "regular" doctor who suggested that she spend several thousand dollars on CT scans and an MRI. She decided a more conservative opinion should be considered, so here she was. During the first visit she told me that she knew all about older women and osteoporosis. She knew that wasn't her problem, she said, "because I drink lots of milk."

Oh boy, I could just imagine how much fun this was going to be, telling my milk story to someone who "knew" all about osteoporosis.

Believe it or not, she successfully abstained from dairy products for four days, and surprisingly, felt better. She returned for her third visit ten days after her first visit. Her back was "Okay", she reported, but she had experienced two headaches since her second visit. She was upset because she never got headaches before. She had one headache on 4/18 that lasted all day. She had another one on 4/22. She had "only a little bit" of neopolitan ice cream on 4/17, and some cheese on 4/21. Each exposure to casein, the only ones in 10 days, were followed by headaches the following day. I suggested that these two headaches were most likely reactions to casein.

"Well, if my back pain is caused by dairy products, why did I get a headache?"

"I don't know." Sorry. There is so much about the whole phenomenon that I don't know. I have no qualms about saying that, that is, that "I don't know." But, I'm learning more every day. Right now I don't know the answer to that question.

But I'll find out.

Edna called me on 4/24 complaining of an intense headache that began at 1:30 pm. I wasn't able to return her call for two hours. When I did, she explained that she was in a panic, at first, then did her own investigation. When I called her she said the headache was almost gone.

"What did you eat for lunch?" I asked.

"Well, I checked that out. I had a Swanson's™ chicken pot pie."

"Oh no," I said. I was about to continue, but she interrupted.

"I dug the box out of the trash, and it has 'non-fat dry milk' in it. You were right."

I decided not to go on with what I was about to say. My mistake.

I told my wife the story that night. She said, "Swanson's™ pot pie? Did you tell her?"

"No. I decided I'd break the news to her on her next visit."

Did I lose you? What am I talking about, anyway? Swanson's™ pot pie contains an additive that is the second most common cause of headaches. Second only to casein. That substance is a flavor enhancer called monosodium glutamate, MSG. It is found in many packaged foods and is most infamous for its use in Oriental Foods. The next chapter will star MSG.

Unfortunately, I decided to tell this patient about MSG on her next visit, 4/26. She called on the morning of 4/25 after waking up with a severe headache. She and her husband had gone out to dinner on the evening of 4/24, just several hours after I had spoken with her, to a Chinese restaurant. This exacerbation, her headache, was due to another poison, monosodium glutamate (MSG).

So why did she now react to MSG after eliminating dairy products, when she didn't before?

A possible explanation could be a synopsis of the work performed by Hans Selye in the 1930's. He theorized that the body responds to any stress in the same way, whether the stressor is an allergen, a poison, cold weather, fear, etc. He called this response the Generalized Adaptation Syndrome (GAS). He said the response takes place in three phases:

1) **The alarm reaction.** In this stage, the acute symptoms occur after exposure to the stressor, like a headache after a glass of milk.

2) **The stage of resistance.** This stage is similar to Randolph's masking idea. Even though the body is still being exposed to the stressor, it has somehow managed to adapt. Symptoms are very mild during this stage, maybe even unnoticeable.

3) **The stage of exhaustion.** When exposure to the stressor continues, the resistance finally fails, and chronic symptoms take over. Repeated exposure at this stage will progress into more serious disease processes, and eventually to death.

So in some cases, many stressors must be removed to alleviate symptoms. Some people have used dairy products their entire lives. Then one day, their backs give out after lifting a refrigerator. This physical stress caused the alarm reaction, severe pain due to physical damage to ligamentous structures. Relief from symptoms requires removal of all stressors: drop the refrigerator, get physical therapy and chiropractic manipulation, and eliminate dairy products.

The body is like a wagon. The wagon is loaded beyond it's capacity until the axle breaks. The refrigerator was the last thing loaded on the wagon when it broke. But in order to repair the axle, the entire wagon must be unloaded.

Another patient, a 40 year old female, Susan, consulted me because she had chronic neck and shoulder tightness. On her first visit I established a dietary connection, adjusted her neck and upper back, and gave her instructions to avoid all dairy products. She did. She returned in three days with severe low back pain. She had never experienced low back pain before. It lasted for one day and was gone. Her neck and upper back pain was resolved. I consider that her episode of low back pain was due to withdrawal from casein. This sort of withdrawal, however, is rare. Typical withdrawal usually involves a headache, or an overall feeling of lousiness. Intense lower back pain can happen as a result of withdrawal, but is rare.

During the first 30 days of treatment, thorough dietary questioning must take place on every visit. I watch for reactions, or lack of reactions to casein and other poisons to establish the entire cause of the patient's complaints. 95% of cases are resolved with the elimination of casein. Many cases react to MSG, and still other cases go on and on into other causitve agents in the diet, and elsewhere.

One of the most useful tools in managing these cases is a diet diary. The patient keeps a log of all foods eaten, time of day, each day, and a chronological report of symptoms. This tool will cover for poor memory, and will help establish reaction time and expose other possible problem foods.

I've told you what I know about milk and dairy products causing back pain. The specific symptoms will be discussed later. Next, other poisons and allergens.

Questions Designed to Establish Use of Casein

Do you drink coffee?

Black, or cream and sugar?

What do you use for cream?

Do you drink tea?

Straight?

Do you drink milk? (Some people will respond "No, I'm allergic to milk.")

How often, in an average week do you have milk?

Do you use it on cereal?

How often, in an average week, do you have cereal?

What kind of milk do you use?

Do you eat cheese? This includes on and in foods and by itself.

Do you eat Mexican food?

Italian food?

Do you eat yogurt or cottage cheese?

How often, in an average week, do you eat yogurt or cottage cheese?

Cream cheese?

Sour cream?

Do you eat baked potatoes?

What do you put on them?

No Milk

Do you eat salads?
How often?
What kind of dressing do you use?
Do you use butter or margarine?
Do you eat ice cream?
How often in an average week?
Do you eat chocolate?
How often?
Are you on any kind of a special diet?
Let's go through a typical day in your diet.
What do you have for breakfast? Lunch? Dinner?
Do you like to eat out?
If so, where?
What did you have for supper last night?
What did you have for lunch today or yesterday?
And on and on and on.

3

Beyond Milk:
Other Allergens
and Poisons

The state of American health is in sad shape due to the Standard American Diet (SAD). Heart disease is the number one killer in this country. Viral infections are increasing. New ones, like AIDS are popping up every day, and most of them have no cure. Arthritis is so common that it has become a way of life in our country. As a result, walkers and wheel chairs are being mass-produced, and handicapped parking spaces are everywhere. Four point walkers can be picked up at garage sales after Aunt Ethel has finally died, or become confined to bed. Americans can be seen everywhere, dragging around their oxygen tanks with the clear plastic tubes draped over their ears and into their noses. Kids are tripping over them in the aisles of the local greasy spoon, where their owners are sitting, hooked to the other end, tanking up on more Standard American crap.

Visit a hospital sometime. See the emphysema patient, all dressed in green, dragging the pole stand with the swinging IV bottle, down the hall to the smoking area where he can put a lighter to his head, then suck the tar and nicotine into his lungs through his tracheotomy.

My wife is from Holland. Her vision of America was created by the American fashion magazines she "wished" through as a young girl. American women are so thin and rich, she thought. American men are so virile and athletic, it seemed. She was shocked when she finally got here and saw how Americans really looked. The athlete of the year is George Foreman!?

The American Cancer Society is throwing billions of dollars at the dreaded "C word" every year for research, but the dying American public keeps throwing it back to the doctors and hospitals and insurance companies. What a waste of money. We know what causes cancer. It's SAD, isn't it?

Yes. It's SAD. The Standard American Diet is one of the main causes of cancer. The Standard American Diet is the main cause of disease in this country. This book is about back pain, neck pain, and headaches that are caused by specific substances in the Standard American Diet. The main cause of these symptoms, as was discussed in the last chapter, is casein, the protein found in milk and dairy products. Americans think milk is health food. However, there are many other substances, allergens and poisons, that can also cause these symptoms.

In cases of neck pain, back pain, and headaches, casein is the number one cause. Undisputed second place goes to mono-sodium glutamate, MSG. Many people are aware of MSG. Many people know that it causes some problems for some people. The American public is becoming more and more aware each year of the health hazards in the Standard American Diet, but almost none of these people are aware of how often and where MSG appears in their foods.

About 75% of the patients I see are aware of what MSG is, that is, they have HEARD of it. Most of them have heard just enough to be able to butcher the name, "MSG? Yeah, mono gluta sodium something or other...?"

"Yeah, I know about MSG. Yeah, that stuff is real bad. I know I can't eat that stuff, wow, it makes me real sick! Me and my husband, we NEVER have that stuff! We can't! If we eat Chinese food, we get really sick. We make sure when we go out that they don't use MSG! We tell em!"

I can usually ask these people a few questions that will reveal that they ate MSG within the last 24 hours. It's not their fault. They are not ignorant or stupid. They are victims of a huge conspiracy. They have been duped, mislead by experts.

That's about the extent of the average American's knowledge of MSG, except they think it's a preservative. Almost all new health food books mention it. I always check out the newest health food, or diet books on the book shelves at the book store. I always thumb directly to the index and look for two things: milk and MSG. Milk is usually listed as the best source of dietary calcium. Most of the time, there is one entry for MSG, page 87, and several entries for milk. If the author mentions MSG on only one or two pages, I have learned that he or she knows about it, but probably agrees with the rest of the "scientific community:"

"MSG is an additive found in many foods and is thought to cause problems in certain, sensitive individuals. But scientific evidence is inconclusive about establishing MSG as a health hazard."

You know, if I still worked in a warehouse, there is only one word for this "analysis" by the scientific community and any individual who claims to be a health expert. This word can be found all over the stockyard floors of America, and at the rodeos, and these "health experts" should be out there shoveling it up, and not into their books and "studies."

I don't work in a warehouse anymore, so I won't say it, but I still know it when I see it. If I see a health book that devotes a whole page to MSG, I know when I turn to that page I will read some innocuous statement that shows me this expert is simply not aware of the extent of the problems caused by MSG. It's a lot like the milk connection: if you don't look, you won't see it. Then when you do, you're surprised at how obvious it seems.

An eyes open, clinical experience by a knowledgeable clinician will reveal the real truth about MSG. A true accounting of MSG, where it is, who uses it, and what it does, will appear in a true treatise on several pages, or a whole chapter, and will initiate law suits, or at least blushes from those manufacturers who use it. Here goes:

The most thorough and honest accounting of MSG appears in a book by George Schwartz, M.D. The name of his book is, *In Bad Taste — The MSG Syndrome.*

I have only just begun to look for the problems caused by MSG in the last two years. That's when I ordered Dr. Schwartz's book after stumbling across an ad for it in a health magazine. I didn't just read his book, then believe him. I read his book, then opened my eyes and started paying attention. As each day passes, I am learning that the MSG problem is a bigger monster than even Dr. Schwartz has portrayed. Read this book and you will never eat out again. This chapter is a synopsis of that book, and my clinical experience with MSG, arguably the single biggest health hazard and health conspiracy in this country.

MSG is not a preservative, as most people think. MSG is a flavor enhancer that is found in most packaged foods, almost all canned or packaged soups, TV dinners, most brands of tuna fish, bacon, lunch meats, many spices, sauces, in fast food restaurants, in fancy restaurants, in Chinese Foods, in many "natural" foods, and on and on. MSG, when added to foods, causes the flavor of the other ingredients to become "amplified."

MSG was first isolated from seaweed in 1908. It was patented in 1909 as a flavor enhancer. It was produced in the orient as Aji-no-moto and distributed by a company of the same name. By 1933 this company was producing 10 million pounds a year. It wasn't until 1948 that MSG was introduced successfully into this country. Food manufacturers were so impressed with it, that it caught on like wildfire. It's use grew unbelievably. It wasn't until 1968 that people started to become aware of possible bad reactions to the substance.

An article appeared in the *New England Journal of Medicine* in 1968 by a Dr. Ho Man Qwok. He had noticed his reaction to Chinese food, which he described as "numbness at the back of the neck gradually radiating to both arms and the back, and general weakness and palpitation." His work received a lot of rebuke, and he was dubbed "Dr. Qwack."

Since that time, the awareness in the medical professions and the public of the ill effects of MSG has grown. But this increasing awareness couldn't possibly quell the fervor of its users. It makes food taste great. It makes some people crave its taste. And because of these attributes, it turns a huge profit by directly increasing food sales.

I think America is the greatest country in the world. I think the free enterprise system is the best economic system in the world. But, it has its weaknesses. When the motivation to provide a good product or service is rewarded with money, some people lose track of their motivation to provide quality goods and services, and become motivated instead by the money. They end up cutting corners to save costs, or they participate in harmful practices because they turn a better profit. Does a doctor order expensive tests and x-rays because the information is important? Or is it because it costs more, putting more money into a clinic, or his or her pocket? Or does it protect him from a lawsuit? Or is it because insurance companies will pay for them?

Do food manufacturers put harmful ingredients in their products because it increases the shelf life, makes it look better, or make it taste better so sales and profits are increased?

Yes. It's SAD, isn't it?

The American public is becoming increasingly aware of the many poisons in our foods. Many people know about MSG. But food manufacturers still want to provide a tasty product that will sell, sell, sell. They know that duplicating the flavor enhancement of MSG using natural herbs and spices would be costly. The flavor provided by these natural herbs and spices would not have the "addictive" quality of MSG. Yes, like other poisons and allergens, MSG can become addictive. I have had many patients report that they "crave" Chinese food.

Food manufacturers have learned to operate around the labelling guidelines of the FDA, so they can continue to use MSG — even though they know it's poison.

A label on any packaged foods lists the ingredients in order of quantity of the ingredient: the first ingredient listed makes up the greatest percentage of ingredients, and the last one makes up the smallest portion. However, certain ingredients, that contain many subingredients, can be listed with no mention of what they contain. "Hydrolyzed Vegetable Protein," (HVP), for example, appears on many labels. HVP contains as much as 20% MSG. HVP can also appear on labels as "Hydrolyzed Plant Protein," or "hydrolyzed protein," or "protein hydrolysate." So if these words appear on labels, that food contains MSG without actually admitting it.

Most canned tuna fish contains MSG. It is usually listed as "hydrolyzed protein." Starkist™ lists three ingredients on its Chunk Light Tuna in water: Tuna, vegetable broth, and water. Most packaged soups and broths contain MSG. I called the consumer information person at Starkist™ and asked if the tuna or the broth contained MSG. I was told that it didn't. However, when I sent the tuna to a lab to be tested, the results were positive for MSG.

Many packaged foods will list an ingredient called "natural flavors," or "natural flavorings." The FDA defines "natural flavorings" as: "the essential oil, oleoresin, essence or extractive, **protein hydrolysate**, distillate or any product of roasting, heating or enzymolysis which contains the flavoring constituents derived from a spice, fruit or fruit juice, vegetable or vegetable juice, edible yeast, herb, bark, root, leaf or similar plant material, meat, seafood, poultry, eggs, **dairy products** or fermentation products thereof whose significant function in food is flavoring rather than nutritional."

Beyond Milk: Other Allergens and Poisons

In this book, I've mentioned the reactions people have to MSG and dairy products, both of which can be included in "natural flavorings." Look at all the other ingredients that could have serious consequences for people who are sensitive to, say eggs, or yeast. Everyone is being mislead by this kind of labelling. It seems that food labelling, initially designed to inform people, has been twisted around by food manufacturers to mislead people.

MSG is a flavor enhancer that adds a very zesty, full, delicious flavor to any dish to which it is added. When added to canned soups, the "tinny" taste of the can magically disappears, so you'll find it in almost all Campbell's™ Soups, Progresso™ Soups, Anderson™ Soups, and almost any other brand of canned soup. You'll find it in the packaged soups, too: Cup a' Soup™, Cup o' Noodles™, Top Ramen™. Most restaurants use MSG in their soups. Most sauce mixes use MSG. You'll find it in most lunch meats, hot dogs, bacon, chorizo, and sausages. Many brands of tuna fish use MSG, like Chicken of the Sea™, Bumble Bee™, Geisha™, and Starkist™. Many restaurants use MSG, or Accent, in sauces, soups, and in many of their "tastiest" dishes. Guess what one of Colonel Sander's secret herbs and spices is in his Kentucky Fried Chicken™? MSG. It is used in most breadings on meats and onion rings.

Many TV dinners use MSG to enhance the flavor that has been dulled by freezing. Many diet programs, like Jenny Craig™ and Weight Watchers™, that use packaged dinners, use MSG. I once saw a patient who began having severe headaches shortly after starting on a diet program. I asked her to bring in some empty boxes of some of the products she was using. Almost all of them used HVP. In fact, most of the dishes had HVP listed two and three times on the label. When she reported to her "diet counselor" that I had instructed her to stop using their products, the counselor called me. She was upset and wanted to know why. I told her that her products contained MSG. She told me that she was "absolutely certain" that they used no MSG.

I referred her to several sources to become more informed. I never heard from her again, although I continue to advise my patients to avoid her diet program. Even though she was supposedly informed about her product, she was left in the dark by the manufacturer. I'm sure she believed her products had no MSG, but she was mislead, and wrong. She has become a puppet of the manufacturer, probably informing curious clients, and with sincere conviction, that they can "rest assured" they are not eating MSG. "Look. Do you see it on the label?"

I am seeing a patient who experiences neck pain and headaches. His case is a complex one. His sensitivities go way beyond dairy products and MSG, although he does react to these two. He has been permanently disabled from work for his psychological problems. He has been arrested several times for severe emotional outbursts of rage. He often becomes distraught and cries uncontrollably for no apparent reason, or at the slightest provocation. He hears voices. His doctors have been managing his case with drugs and psychiatric counseling. Although we are far from totally solving his problems, he is doing very well emotionally by avoiding dairy products and MSG and sugar, and several other suspected allergens. He is doing a superlative job of managing his diet, but, as is sometimes the case, his family finds it annoying. Several weeks ago, he took his family for a ride.

When it was time to eat, his wife suggested Kentucky Fried Chicken™. He ordered for his family, then fell into a quandary about what he could eat. His wife was perturbed. What a pain he was. His wife called for the teenaged "manager" and asked him if they used MSG in their chicken.

"Absolutely not," he responded.

His wife was so perturbed that he decided not to press any further. Within a few minutes of eating the chicken, he became angry. Fortunately, he knew what was happening and managed to get away. His reaction lasted for five days. He came in to see me six days after the MSG reaction caused by the MSG laden Kentucky Fried Chicken™. He was still sobbing uncontrollably, although his rage had ceased.

Beyond Milk: Other Allergens and Poisons

The classic symptoms I have seen in my practice due to exposure to MSG are headaches, irritability, stomach upset, shoulder, neck, and arm pain. Onset of pain is usually much faster than the typical 2 to 12 hour reaction time of allergy to casein. Symptoms begin usually in a few minutes to a few hours after ingesting MSG. As a chiropractor, one of the most interesting symptoms is the neck, shoulder, and arm pain. In most cases, the left side is involved, although it can affect the right side, or both sides. The patient usually complains of severe pain and spasm in the neck, radiating into the arm and down into the shoulder blade. It's almost always on one side only, usually the left. Many times it radiates into the chest. The patient may begin to sweat and experience shortness of breath. Many patients experience a fullness in the throat.

The left sided chest and arm symptoms usually cause extreme alarm to the patient and medical people because it looks a lot like a heart attack. The typical scenario is a scene of panic, an ambulance ride to the nearest hospital, x-rays and an EKG (electro cardiogram). Then the puzzlement. The tests are all negative and the symptoms go away in a few hours. The doctors and patients all shrug and assume it was an anxiety attack of some sort.

Then the weird questions begin, "Are you happy at home?" The most pointed question in any situation like this, of course is, "What did you eat?" I'm sure there are many cases of MSG exposure and reaction that actually proceed to heart attack and death. I wonder about Hank Gathers.

Monosodium glutamate consists of sodium and glutamate. Glutamate is a salt of the amino acid, glutamic acid.. Glutamate acts as an excitatory neurotransmitter. After only 90 seconds of contact, it causes swelling of nerves. Glutamate affects blood vessels in the brain. Our understanding of the brain and nervous system is very poor. Many of the poorly understood diseases are malfunctions of the nervous system: Alzheimer's, Huntington's chorea, Parkinson's disease, Lou Gehrig's disease, multiple sclerosis, and on and on. Recent studies have implicated glutamate toxicity as a possible cause of Alzheimer's Disease and Huntington's chorea. The medical books all list the same cause: unknown. To me, the causes are not going to be found by closely analyzing the tissue changes in these disorders, but to consider poisons and/or allergens that are circulating through the blood. When considering a chemical, I think it is pointless to inject some poor innocent lab animal with a huge dose of the stuff, then analyze its suffering.

Manufacturers removed MSG from baby food in 1969 after "some doubt" about its safety was aroused by the reactions of lab animals to glutamic acid. To assume that reactions in animals are similar to reactions in humans is a questionable assumption that makes animal vivisection a poorly founded "science." But to assume that reactions in animals have some correlation to human infants, but not to other humans is beyond any kind of logic. To get questionable reactions that raise "some doubt" as to the safety of a substance would seem to me to indicate complete removal of the substance from all human consumption. But to come to the conclusion that there is no "real scientific evidence" that MSG is harmful after torturing animals with it, so deciding to leave it on the market while more tests are conducted, is the most ludicrous scientific practice I have ever seen. The animals suffer, people suffer, but we don't want to pull it off the market because doing so might lower profits for some food manufacturers. It makes me wonder what goes on behind closed doors.

Many American women (and their mates) suffer with PMS, premenstrual syndrome. Talk about poorly understood disorders. The workings of the female hormone system are a puzzlement to most practitioners, a bane to marriages and relationships, and an endless source for magazine articles, talk shows, and pharmaceutical products.

Maybe that's because most gynecologists are men. I don't pretend to understand PMS any better, but I do know this: PMS involves a myriad of symptoms including abdominal cramps, headaches, irritability, depression, anxiety, and mood swings in those unfortunate women who suffer from it. These symptoms usually begin a week or a few days before the monthly menstrual flow, and are thought to be due to the hormonal changes of the cycle.

But some women suffer severe symptoms, and others don't suffer at all. The medical approach of the past, and still a big business, is to rip out the source of the hormones: a hysterectomy. Sometimes that works, but so did frontal lobotomies. I think the practice of removing vital organs so a person can act appropriately is ridiculous. We have discussed the fact that substances such as chocolate and MSG can cause PMS type symptoms in some people. Many women crave these substances around their periods, ingest them, then act accordingly. Some of these women don't eat these foods any other time during the month. Some women eat chocolate and MSG at other times of the month, but don't show PMS symptoms then.

So what does all this mean? Well, maybe the hormone changes of the menses cause cravings for substances that cause mood changes. Maybe the menses causes an increased sensitivity to substances that cause mood changes. Whatever the mechanism, it just seems to make more sense to eliminate substances that cause PMS symptoms before more aggressive, irreversible procedures are performed. Maybe a hysterectomy will be necessary after aggressive dietary manipulation with no change in symptoms. But I doubt it.

Monosodium glutamate is a poison that affects all people, some more than others, depending on sensitivity. Poisons are dose dependent, so more MSG will cause more severe symptoms. Some people are also allergic to MSG, and will react with more classic allergy symptoms, like hives. After the casein in milk and dairy products, MSG is the most common substance causing back pain, neck pain, and headaches. Patients who complain of these symptoms will almost always respond after they have eliminated dairy products and all MSG from their diets. I suspect that many allergies, or reactions to substances, are affected by different combinations of substances. I discussed before the combination of an allergen with sugar, making the reaction more intense. I suspect a similar relationship, in many cases, with MSG and casein. It seems that some patients begin reacting to MSG, when they didn't before, after casein has been eliminated from the diet. If this relationship is not considered, case management can become difficult.

If a causal relationship between a patient's symptoms and casein in the diet can be established in the history, the logical course is to instruct the patient to avoid casein. However, I am finding more and more that it is necessary to establish how much MSG is in the diet, then eliminate it too. Many times, we eliminate casein, and the patient gets better, then suffers a recurrence of symptoms after exposure to MSG. After successfully convincing this kind of patient of the milk connection, and now having to explain MSG, my credibility to the patient sometimes seems questionable. The patient begins to believe that a new food will be eliminated every time symptoms recur. So, to save possible trouble, I usually explain and eliminate MSG on the first visit, along with casein.

Eliminating these two substances, one an allergen, one a poison, will solve most cases of neck pain, back pain, and headaches. In fact, **99% of all headaches will be solved by eliminating MSG and casein.** However, eliminating these two substances is just a starting point in some cases. Some people are highly allergenic, and suffer with all kinds of symptoms after exposure to lots of different substances. These cases can become very complex and time consuming. When considering these cases, and others that are less complex, other allergens and poisons must be considered.

A thorough history of symptoms and diet is necessary to provide direction for the case. The symptoms may seem to be classic for allergy to casein, but if it can be established that the patient does not eat dairy products, other substances must be considered. In my experience, the next group of foods to consider is one or more of the common food allergens. A person can become allergic to anything, especially after repeated exposure. Knowing this, it is not difficult to establish that the most common food allergens are the most common foods. Milk and dairy is number one, by far, because it is the most commonly used food in this country. Other common food allergens are wheat, corn, soy, eggs, coffee, and cane sugar.

If symptoms persist after casein and MSG have been eliminated, a diet history will point the way to the next substance to be considered. Usually that is wheat. Allergy, or sensitivity to wheat has been known to the medical profession for many years. The typical symptoms of this sensitivity are digestive. Celiac disease has been recognized for nearly 2000 years, and the early Greeks noticed that bread seemed to aggravate the symptoms. The digestive symptoms in children have been designated as celiac disease, and in adults as sprue. Here again we see the common misconception that a childhood disease that continues into adulthood should be renamed and treated differently.

In 1950, a Dutch pediatrician, Dr. Willem Karel Dicke, reported that sprue and celiac disease were one and the same. He also identified gluten as the causitive agent. Gluten is the protein fraction found in wheat. It is a complex structure with several proteins contributing to its makeup, mainly gliaden, which gives bread its extensibility, and glutenin, which gives bread its elasticity. Dr. Dicke was able to establish that the aggravating agent in gluten is gliadin. When he suggested eliminating wheat from the diet in children who suffered with the digestive symptoms of celiac disease, he was ridiculed. When two other Dutch physicians set out to prove him wrong, they saw the indisputable "wheat connection."

Many times the symptoms of gluten sensitivity are digestive, like upset stomach, irritable bowel, smelly, greasy stools, etc. However, as we have discussed, allergic symptoms are systemic. When the allergen, in this case gluten, is circulating through the blood stream, any system can be affected. Headaches, decreased energy, joint and muscle pain are some of the manifestations of gluten sensitivity. Dr. R. Shatin of Australia has investigated the relationship between gluten intolerance and rheumatoid arthritis and multiple sclerosis (MS). He suggested that the primary lesion of MS is in the small intestine, caused by gluten intolerance, causing the secondary lesion of demyelination of the nerve sheaths. It is my consideration that MS can be a result of any sensitivity or allergy, not just gluten.

The many different symptoms of allergy are due to the fact that the circulating protein can affect any and many systems. The nervous system is involved many times, maybe every time. When the nervous system malfunctions, due to exposure to allergens and/or poisons, the symptoms become seemingly weird to many patients and doctors. Many of these patients are signed off as "head cases," sometimes being diagnosed as character disorders, schizophrenic, manic-depressive, or criminally insane. Dr. Curtis Dohan has seen the connection between behavior disorders and gluten intolerance. He made the connection by observing that children with celiac disease, more often than "by mere chance," became schizophrenic adults, and that psychoses in adult celiacs were also disturbingly common. He completed the bio-ecological puzzle by noting that psychoses were often relieved when these patients were placed on a gluten-free diet.

The following conclusion was reached by M.M. Singh and S.R. Kay after a study at the Bronx Psychiatric Center:

"Schizophrenics maintained on a cereal grain-free and milk-free diet and receiving optimal treatment with neuroleptics showed an interruption or reversal of their therapeutic progress during a 'blind' wheat gluten challenge. The exacerbation of the disease process was not due to the variations in neuroleptic doses. After termination of the gluten challenge, the course of improvement was reinstated. The observed effects seemed to be due to a primary schizophrenic promoting effect of wheat gluten."[1]

Some studies performed in the 1960's in Scandinavia, and Mexico, and elsewhere indicated a possible relationship between gluten intolerance and lactose intolerance. It seems

---

[1] Beatrice Trum Hunter, *Gluten Intolerance,* Keats Publishing, New Canaan, Connecticut, 1987.

that lactose intolerance in infants is often succeeded by gluten intolerance in adults. These studies suggested that gluten intolerance is possibly a sequel to lactose intolerance.

In another study, men who had been diagnosed as infertile, were able to impregnate women after strict adherence to a gluten-free diet. In yet another study, women who had been unable to conceive, became pregnant after avoiding gluten. Case histories of these women revealed a history of celiac disease in childhood. After failing to follow the gluten-free diet, their apparently "masked" symptoms manifested themselves in adulthood as infertility.

Cane sugar is a common allergen. Many parents and teachers are aware of many children's reactions to sugar as hyperactivity, anger, mood changes, drowsiness, etc. When problems continue into adulthood, a common diagnosis is hypoglycemia. This diagnosis has become popular over the last twenty years and is commonly discounted by conventional medics. It seems that, to some doctors, if it wasn't in the medical textbooks in the 1920's, it doesn't exist. When exposure to sugar continues, despite hypoglycemic symptoms, the disease progresses into diabetes.

Many people are aware of their reaction to sugar as an immediate, energized "high," followed by a rapid plunge into fatigue, drowsiness, or depression. The explanation of this phenomenon is a malfunction of sugar metabolism, and dubbed hypoglycemia. Blood sugar, or blood glucose, is maintained at a constant level in the blood stream. Variations in the blood glucose caused by ingestion of carbohydrates (chains of sugar molecules), are detected by the brain and controlled by the pancreas. As the blood glucose begins to rise after a meal, the brain tells the pancreas to secrete insulin into the bloodstream. Insulin "escorts" glucose out of the blood and into the tissue, where it is stored. Glucose is stored in the liver as glycogen. When the blood glucose begins to drop between meals, the stored glycogen is mobilized back into the blood stream to maintain the desirable blood sugar. Ideally, this up and down surge of blood glucose is maintained within normal limits, so the activity level of the individual is a smooth operation. In hypoglycemia, the oscillation of blood glucose is radical.

Glucose is the product of the breakdown of carbohydrates. The simple carbohydrates, found in refined sugar and processed foods, are rapidly broken down into glucose. When these foods are ingested, the blood sugar surges, causing an intense over-reaction by the pancreas. The intense surge of insulin into the blood causes the blood glucose to rapidly plunge below normal. This roller coaster, up and down surge of blood glucose causes the highs and lows of hypoglycemia. In the intense lows, the individual can feel weak, faint, and get the shakes, requiring a sugar "fix" to get back to normal. Whole grains and vegetables are made up of complex carbohydrates, complex molecules that are broken down into glucose more slowly. These natural foods are digested more slowly, giving the blood a steady flow of glucose, the kind of glucose source the pancreas was designed to handle.

Bio ecologists have recognized that the symptoms of hypo-glycemia are similar to the symptoms of allergy. Dr. Philpott has been investigating hypoglycemia, and has discovered that low blood sugar levels can be produced by foods containing little or no carbohydrate. Those darn bio-ecologists! Always stirring up trouble! Dr. Philpott cites a case where a man allergic to milk demonstrated extreme low blood sugar two hours after the ingestion of cream cheese. Cream cheese is only 2% carbohydrate. He concluded: "The assumption that these disordered carbohydrate reactions will be in response to carbohydrate only is not valid. Testing reveals that they occur to any type of food and that the central cause is that of being allergic to or allergic in a specific way to a specific food whether fat, protein or carbohydrate. In this case the hypogly-cemic response was to cream cheese which is largely a protein and fat food."

Dr. H.L. Newbold, a psychiatrist saw his own poor health improve after he changed his diet. He now treats patients using a bio ecology approach, and concludes that he believes **practically all hypoglycemia is the result of allergy.**

Beyond Milk: Other Allergens and Poisons

It has now become a new thought in bio ecology, that the target organ of food allergy, or the first organ affected, is the pancreas. Hypoglycemia, therefor, is not strictly a reaction to carbohydrate metabolism. It is the bio ecologist's point of view that the many supposed hypoglycemics who improved after dietary changes, did so after accidentally eliminating allergenic foods while they were instructed to eliminate only simple carbohydrates.

* The pancreas functions not only in the breakdown of carbohydrates, by secreting insulin, but also by producing enzymes necessary for food metabolism.The failure of the pancreas to produce the enzymes necessary for the breakdown of fats, proteins, and carbohydrates, leaves foods incompletely digested. Instead of amino acids, the basic units of proteins, being absorbed, unusable protein molecules are absorbed and sent circulating in the blood. These proteins cause the release of histamines and kinins, inflammatory reactions, throughout the body, producing the widespread symptoms of allergy. Symptoms will show up in weak tissue and will be diagnosed by conventional medics as some specific disease unrelated to pancreatic dysfunction. In fact, as this new theory goes, all these diseases can be traced back to chemical diabetes mellitus caused by allergens and poisons interfering with metabolic processes.

The definitive work on clinical bio-ecology has been done over the last 25 or so years by Dr. Marshall Mandell. Dr. Mandell has concluded from his studies that **reactive hypoglycemia as a response to excessive consumption of simple carbohydrates may not even exist!**

How did he get away with that? I once suggested to the husband of a women who suffered with lupus erythematosis, that her symptoms could most likely be due to allergy, and perhaps the disease entity of lupus didn't even exist. He misinterpreted my comment to be a denial that his wife was sick, and he cancelled a talk I had been scheduled to deliver to "his" lupus support group. Lupus Erythematosis is another disease entity with multiple system involvement, cause unknown.

It looks like allergy, and most likely is. I did manage to squeeze in one talk to this lupus group before I was banned. I spoke of allergy, and one woman stood up and reported that she did see a severe attack of her symptoms after a glass of milk. I managed to get a dietary questionnaire back from six people in the group. Each of these six people reported that they craved and ate chocolate every day. In fact, after the meeting, one woman, a confessed "chocoholic," told me she would do anything to be rid of her symptoms. When I suggested she should start with giving up chocolate, she said "Anything but that."

Dr. Marshall Mandell's work can be examined in his book, *Dr. Mandell's Five Day Allergy Relief System*. He has elaborated on Dr. Randolph and Dr. Rinkel's practice of four day avoidance of allergens followed by feeding challenges of suspected allergens. Most bio-ecologists practice based on a thorough history designed to determine possible allergens that have caused the patient's complaints. In my practice, which is limited to musculoskeletal and neurological symptoms, I can usually establish one or two or three probable culprits, starting of course with milk and dairy and MSG. Most cases are solved right here with these two aggravating agents being eliminated. Some cases proceed beyond this point, as I have discussed. When other substances must be considered, like wheat or sugar, a further, more accurate history can be accumulated by the patient using a diet diary. Using this tool, the patient writes down each day what foods were eaten, the time of day they were eaten, and a chronological accounting of symptoms. If a patient considers that any symptom can be, and usually is due to allergy, and any food can cause symptoms, a long term diet diary will enlighten them about how much they are what they eat. When they pay attention long enough, they will proceed way beyond the milk connection, especially when they consider physical discomfort, mood changes, energy level, etc.

Dr. Mandell is aggressive and opinionated. He's my hero. In his practice, he sees many, many more symptoms than I do. He looks for his best guesses when interviewing the patient, then makes recommendations accordingly. Many cases, however, are very complex, and simple connections are sometimes impossible to make. In these cases, he recommends a five day water fast where all foods are eliminated. He contends that, if a patient's symptoms are due to food allergy, a five day fast, where the patient drinks only purified water, will cause symptoms to abate. After the five day fast, the patient is fed different foods, best guesses first, in an allergy challenge. Reactions are observed. Symptom producing foods are eliminated from the diet.

After reading his book in 1988, I fasted for five days, to see if it could be done, and how difficult it was. I managed it, with some difficulty. I felt hungry on day one and day two, tired on day three, and better, with no hunger on day four. On day five I felt like superman, lots of energy, clear headed, no hunger. It can be done, but I've recommended it to patients only twice. Neither patient was able to make it past day two. But I must consider the difficulty for them, since they suffered with complex symptoms, and undoubtedly experienced more intense withdrawal than I had.

In my clinical experience, expecting symptoms that are due to food allergy to completely abate after five days of avoidance, is pushing it. I have seen cases of seven day withdrawal many times, and several cases that went longer before symptoms changed. Now, maybe I was missing something, maybe the patient was still inadvertently being exposed to the allergen, I don't know. These possibilities were explored with questioning, but, as I've pointed out, there are plenty of holes in even the most thorough investigative approach, considering memory, honesty, etc. But, to be conservative, I recommend avoidance of suspected allergens for a full thirty days.

Any food can be an allergen. After considering milk, then MSG, then wheat, a thorough history and diet diary must lead the way into the consideration of other possible allergens for chronic problems. The aggravating agent in a one time, acute reaction can many times be isolated with a thorough history. But to determine the allergen in a chronic complaint, a regularly used food must be considered.

Corn is a common food allergen because of its heavy use in the American diet. Corn syrup is used in soft drinks and other foods as a sweetener. Corn oil is widely used and a common ingredient in margarine. Overexposure can cause a sensitivity to develop, manifesting itself as any of the aforementioned systemic disorders, very commonly as joint pain.

Soy is another food allergen to be considered. It is commonly used in this country. Unfortunately, most casein free milk substitutes are made with soy. If a milk sensitive patient substitutes soy milk, and uses it regularly, allergy to soy may develop. I once saw a 26 year old woman who suffered from headaches. They began six months prior to her visit to my office, shortly after she began taking vitamins. After two months of suffering, she increased her vitamins. Her headaches became worse. She had also changed her diet and was eating tofu and taking lecithen, both soy products. When I examined her vitamins, I saw that many of them contained soy. My best guess, based on the above, was that soy was the aggravating agent. I instructed her to stop taking vitamins and tofu and lecithen, all soy. Pretty weird health advice, huh? Well, her headaches stopped. So did a skin rash that had concurrently developed around her finger nails. Soy allergy.

Many health conscious people are turning to vegetarian diets. In my opinion, eliminating animal products from the diet is probably the single most powerful health inducing dietary change a person can make. However, many vegetarian programs rely on soy products heavily. Soy allergy can commonly result.

Nightshade vegetables must be considered as aggravating agents in some cases. Members of this group of vegetables include tomatoes, potatoes, egg plant, and peppers of all kinds, red and green bell peppers, cayenne, chili, paprika, etc. (not white or black pepper). Other members of the nightshade group include many powerful stimulating, poisonous, or medicinal plants, like tobacco, henbane, mandrake, and belladona. Nightshade vegetables were first used by the Incas, but initially thought to be poisonous in Europe. Eventually, potatoes became popular and replaced grain as the staple food in northern Europe. Tomatoes became popular in southern Europe.

Nightshades are high in alkaloids, denatured proteins that have a powerful effect on the nervous system. They can act as stimulants, hallucinogens, and medicines (uh oh). Other well known alkaloids include caffeine, theobromine (in chocolate), opium, morphine, heroin, strychnine, quinine, nicotine, atropine, belladonna, and scopalomine. Cattle grazing on the nightshade *Solanum malacoxylon* grew sick, suffered from arthritis, and ended up grazing on their knees. They suffered from excess calcium and phosphorus in the blood, leading to calcium deposits in the aorta, kidneys, lungs, and neck. Animal studies.

In human studies, I once saw a 48 year old man that complained of neck stiffness that radiated into his left shoulder. He had just begun gardening, and tomatoes were growing like weeds. He was eating them in salads every day. When he eliminated them, his symptoms stopped.

Another patient I saw had suffered with headaches, low back pain, and right leg pain that was due to allergy to casein. When dairy products were eliminated, he recovered and was released. After he began analyzing his diet further, he dropped by one day to tell me that he experienced neck and shoulder spasms after eating tomato products like catsup, and tomato sauce. However, he claimed, he did not react to raw tomatoes. This, to me, is an indicator that some allergens produce symptoms only when combined with other substances, like perhaps sugar.

Beyond food allergies lie the poisons. I must be quite frank here. I have studied the relationships between certain foods and certain symptoms. It has taken me six years to put together the milk connection. Much work remains. Over the last two years, I have taken notice of MSG and its effects on many people. I have seen and read that other foods can cause similar reactions in people. I believe that cancer research is way off target, a waste of money. I know what causes cancer — it's the same thing that causes most disease: allergens and poisons.

And oh, those poisons. I haven't even begun to go beyond reading labels, checking out substances like BHT (butylated hydroxytoluene), BHA (butylated hydroxyanisole), hydroxyquinoline sulfate, nitrates, nitrites, dioxin, potassium bromate, sodium bisulfite, and on and on. What is all that stuff, anyway? It's poison, that's what. I could start to consider the symptoms that some people suffer after exposure to these unnatural substances. I could take notes, manipulate labels, watch for reactions, pick and choose, etc. It would take me years to make specific connections, and I'd probably be wrong half the time. But why bother?

I just have to consider what Hippocrates said before we got so smart, so technical. **"The key to health is through natural living."** Thank God for that. Boy, that saves me a lot of time and trouble. So I know not to eat something that I can't pronounce, or something that has a bunch of x's or y's in its name, or wasn't in the dictionary ten years ago, or is currently being investigated, or is classified by the FDA and the AMA as GRAS (Generally Regarded as Safe).

GRAS=Unsafe for Human Consumption

One of the biggest problems in our country today is the impotent approach our government has taken to the poisoning of our food. The AMA and the FDA conduct studies. They are so scientific, so thorough. They decide that studies are inconclusive. They can't decide how much of a poison a rat or a dog or a monkey can take before it suffers horribly and dies. Based on that indecision, they leave poisons on the market so we can torture more animals, witness more death and disease among humans, and wonder why, and observe in unfeeling silence, before we can accurately conclude that we screwed up, and some food manufacturer is going to have to sacrifice a little bit, or a lot, of profit.

Someone, a lot of someones, are going to have to go out of business for what they have done to those who don't want to rock the boat, or be RUDE at parties, or be fanatics.

Beyond Milk: Other Allergens and Poisons

You want to die?

Then don't care. They'll poison you, take your money, your life savings, and tell you they saved your life. It's a conspiracy. Some overweight, bespectacled doctor is going to tell you, in his expert opinion, that Nutrasweet™ is okay, harmless, a great substitute for regular sugar.

Wrong, wrong, wrong.

Aspartame (Nutrasweet™) is 100 to 200 times sweeter than sugar. The FDA approved aspartame in 1974, then found out it caused brain damage in animals. Later, they took it back and decided it was okay. Sounds fishy to me. In 1984 the Arizona Department of Health Services issued a report that excessive heat cause the aspartame in soft drinks to break down and produce dangerous levels of methyl alcohol. The FDA checked it out and said don't worry. The FDA has received over 4000 reports of adverse reactions to aspartame. That doesn't seem like a lot, but those are the few people who noticed and made the connection.

Aspartame will go the way of all the chemical poisons that can't bribe their way to total annihilation of the human race in the name of health, or good looks, or some other lie. Oh, we'll lose a few people, but the good, caring health care professionals will study the reactions and write books about what aspartame is doing to those who use it.

I prefer to not find out.

Sometimes a poison isn't in the food, but involved in the making or serving of the food. Dioxin is used in some pesticides and in the process of chlorine bleaching of paper plates, coffee filters, and tea bags. Some paper mills dump it into rivers where it was found to cause cancer in fish. What can it do to us? Again, I prefer not to find out, if I can help it. Is it in our drinking water? Unbleached coffee filters and paper products are now available.

When a person is sick, complaining of symptoms that affect multiple systems throughout the body, I first consider that a chemical irritant, an allergen or a poison, is coursing through the blood stream. The blood stream is the supply system for all the tissue of the body. The tissue receives nutrients via the blood stream. The tissue disposes of waste via the blood stream. Without the blood supply, tissue would die. Lack of blood to an area of the brain, cerebrovascular accident, or stroke, causes muscles and organs controlled by that part of the brain to fail. Lack of blood to a part of the heart muscle, myocardial infarct (MI), causes angina (chest pain) or heart failure. The blood stream goes everywhere. Poke yourself with a pin sometime.

When a person complains of symptoms in multiple systems, the typical medical practice is to involve multiple doctors: a specialist for each system. It seems that modern medical practitioners think that the systems of the human body work independently, and are somehow not related to each other. So when a patient consults a general practitioner because he is suffering with headaches, a skin rash, back pain, fatigue, mood swings, and painful urination, the medical circus begins. The general practitioner orders tests, then refers to the orthopedist, who orders tests, who refers to the dermatologist, who orders tests, who refers to the psychiatrist, who orders even more tests, and on and on and on. The test results are sent from this doctor to that doctor and all over the place. Some are lost, some never get there, some are never read. Each doctor prescribes some medication, many times without checking with the other doctors. These patients are now overmedicated, side effects to the drugs further complicate the case. What a mess.

Many patients tell me, "Whenever my back hurts, I get a headache and an upset stomach. Does the back problem cause the headache?

"Or, do I get sick to my stomach because of the pain? Or do I get irritable from the pain? What causes what? And what is the main problem?"

To me, all the complaints are symptoms. The back pain did not cause the headache or the stomach pain or vice versa. But something caused all of the symptoms. Something went into the body, then into the bloodstream, then into the tissues of the body, causing some sort of reaction in those tissues, that caused the symptoms. Yeah, but a high tech blood test shows a chemical in the blood that indicated arthritis! To me, these chemical indicators in the blood, like RA factor, are just other symptoms of reactions.

So to treat each symptom as a separate disorder is missing the point, missing the cause. If the cause is not determined, then eliminated, the case will not be solved by medical intervention.

Fortunately, the human body is perfectly capable of healing itself, despite what the doctors do. I think that's why there are so many medical specialties that get credit for successful treatment. When a patient consults a general practitioner, then begins the musical chair routine of specialists, many times they get better somewhere along the way. Whoever they are seeing at the time gets the credit. Maybe the specialist's intervention stopped the disease, maybe God did. Maybe that's why some people and doctors are confused as to who is who.

Benjamin Franklin defined a doctor as, "The person who takes the fee after God cures."

When a person is sick with multiple system involvement, look to the blood. The blood is affected by what goes into the body, that is, what is breathed in or eaten or absorbed through the skin. When a person is sick, look first to the diet. Most of the answers will be found here and will make any aggressive medical intervention totally unnecessary.

When the dietary cause of disease is eliminated, so will the disease. Sometimes the damage done by eating or breathing poisons and allergens becomes irreversible. For example, scientific tests have finally concluded that cigarette smoking causes emphysema. If you quit smoking, your chances of eventually suffering from emphysema are greatly reduced. But sometimes heavy smokers quit before they get emphysema, but end up getting it several years later anyway. The damage has been done.

No Milk

The bottom line is, like we've all heard for years, "you are what you eat." I like to go to the grocery store, examine the contents of a basket, then look at the driver. Try it sometime. You'll see what we are doing to ourselves.

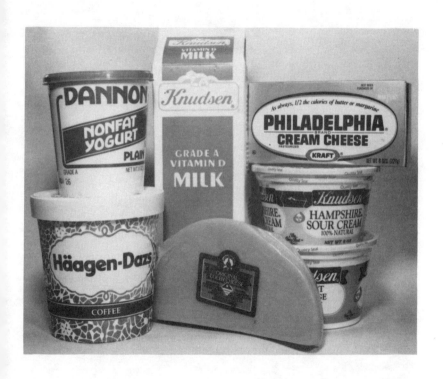

These are the common milk and dairy products Americans know and love. Dairy products are those foods made with cow's milk. Included here is milk, cheese, ice cream, cottage cheese, cream cheese, and yogurt. Eggs are not pictured here because eggs are not dairy products.

145

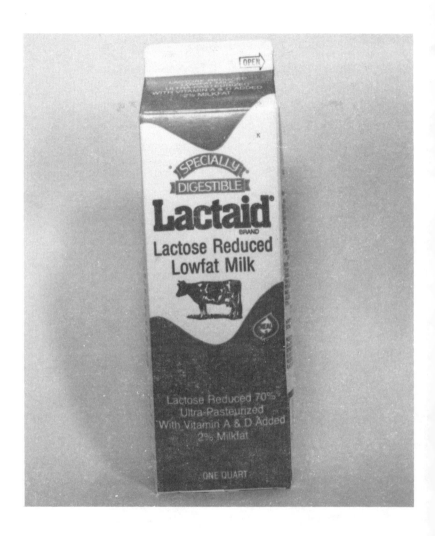

Lactaid™ milk was produced for those people who suffer from lactose intolerance, the inability to digest lactose, the milk sugar. This is cow's milk with lactase enzyme added. This product is still cow's milk, it contains casein, the milk protein, and will cause a reaction in those people who are allergic to milk.

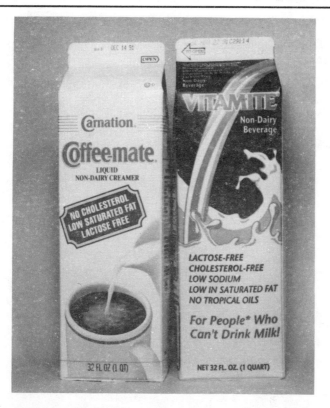

INGREDIENTS: WATER, CORN SYRUP SOLIDS, PARTIALLY HYDROGENATED CANOLA OIL, POTASSIUM CASEINATE (MILK PROTEIN DERIVATIVE), ISOLATED SOY PROTEIN, TRICALCIUM PHOSPHATE, DIPOTASSIUM PHOSPHATE, CARRAGEENAN, SALT, MONO AND DIGLYCERIDES, SODIUM STEAROYL LACTYLATE, GUAR GUM, VITAMIN A PALMITATE, VITAMIN D₃, ANNATTO (COLOR).

Here are two non-dairy creamers in liquid form. They are lactose free, cholesterol free, and low in saturated fat. Although these products are suitable for sufferers of lactose intolerance, they will still cause a reaction in those who are sensitive to the protein, casein. Each label lists "sodium caseinate (a milk derivative)".

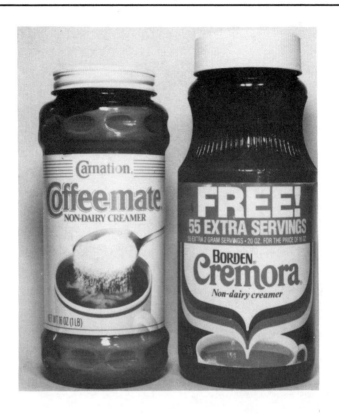

CONTAINS LESS THAN 2% OF THE U.S. RDA OF PROTEIN, VITAMIN A, VITAMIN C, THIAMINE, RIBOFLAVIN, NIACIN, CALCIUM, AND IRON.

INGREDIENTS: CORN SYRUP SOLIDS, PARTIALLY HYDROGENATED VEGETABLE OIL (MAY CONTAIN ONE OR MORE OF THE FOLLOWING OILS—COCONUT, COTTONSEED, PALM, PALM KERNEL, SAFFLOWER, OR SOYBEAN), SODIUM CASEINATE (A MILK DERIVATIVE), MONO- AND DIGLYCERIDES (PREVENT OIL SEPARATION), DIPOTASSIUM PHOSPHATE (MODERATES COFFEE ACIDITY), ARTIFICIAL FLAVOR, AND ANNATTO COLOR.

Here are two powdered non-dairy creamers commonly used at the office coffee station and in some restaurants. These two products also contain sodium caseinate, and will therefor cause a reaction in those who are allergic to the milk protein, casein.

148

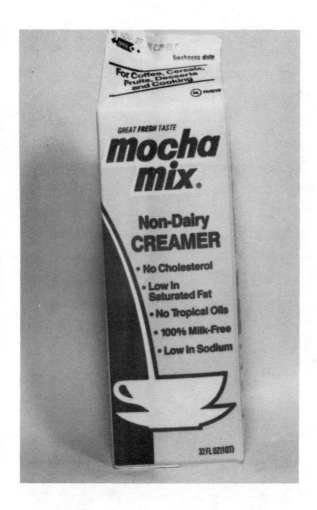

This product is a non-dairy creamer made from soy. It contains no casein or sodium caseinate and is safe for those people who are allergic to casein. Mocha Mix™ contains lots of artificial ingredients, so it is not the healthiest food on the planet. It is man's best attempt to duplicate the taste of cow's milk—a poor attempt. Mocha Mix™ tastes much different than cow's milk, but some people love it. It is thick like cream and may be diluted with water to achieve the desired thickness and taste.

149

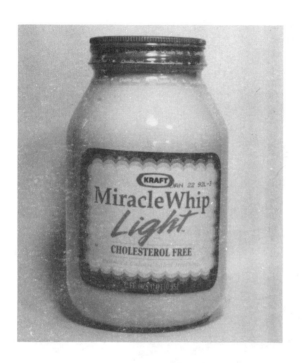

INGREDIENTS: WATER, SOYBEAN OIL, SUGAR, VINEGAR, FOOD STARCH-MODIFIED, SALT, STARCH, CELLULOSE GEL (MICRO-CRYSTALLINE CELLULOSE), SODIUM CASEINATE, MUSTARD FLOUR, EGG WHITE, XANTHAN GUM, SPICE, PAPRIKA, NATU-RAL FLAVOR, BETA CAROTENE (COLOR)

This diet mayonaise contains sodium caseinate and will cause a reaction in those people who are allergic to casein. Regular mayonaise is milk free.

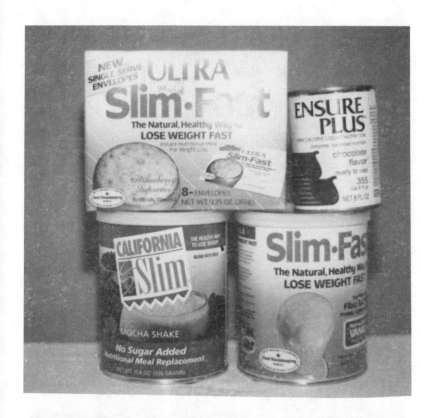

INGREDIENTS: ⑪-D WATER, CORN SYRUP, SUCROSE, CORN OIL, SODIUM AND CALCIUM CASEINATES, COCOA POWDER, SOY PROTEIN ISOLATE, MAGNESIUM CHLORIDE, POTASSIUM CITRATE, CALCIUM PHOSPHATE TRIBASIC, SOY LECITHIN, SODIUM CITRATE, POTASSIUM CHLORIDE, CHOLINE CHLORIDE, ASCORBIC ACID, NATURAL AND ARTIFICIAL FLAVOR, ZINC SULFATE, XANTHAN GUM, FERROUS SULFATE, ALPHA-TOCOPHERYL ACETATE, NIACINAMIDE,

These diet products all contain milk or sodium caseinate or calcium caseinate.

151

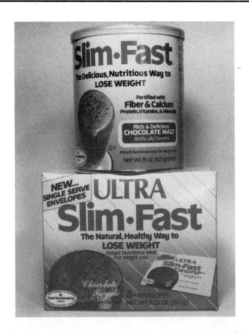

INGREDIENTS: Sucrose, Nonfat Dry Milk, Whey Powder, Purified Cellulose, Soy Protein Isolate, Corn Bran, Whey Protein Concentrate, Fructose, Maltodextrin, Carrageenan, Guar Gum, Lecithin, Citric Acid, DL-Methionine, **Aspartame and, Natural and Artificial Flavor and Color; and the following vitamins and minerals: Calcium Phosphate, Magnesium Oxide, Potassium Chloride, Ferric Orthophosphate, Ascorbic Acid, Vitamin E Acetate, Niacinamide, Vitamin A Palmitate, Zinc Oxide, Manganese Sulfate, Calcium Pantothenate, Copper Sulfate, Vitamin D_3, Pyridoxine Hydrochloride, Thiamine Mononitrate, Riboflavin, Folic Acid, Biotin, Potassium Iodide, Vitamin B_{12}.
**Phenylketonurics: Contains Phenylalanine   A 1668-01

Slim Fast™ and Ultra Slim Fast™ are diet protein drinks that are very popular. Both are to be mixed with low fat or skim milk. Even without the added milk, each product contains milk as the second item on the label. Slim Fast™ also contains calcium caseinate. Many people who suffer with back pain due to allergy to casein begin suffering several days or weeks after starting on a Slim Fast™ diet. To further aggravate their pain, most people choose chocolate flavored Slim Fast™. Of all the foods that cause back pain or headaches, chocolate is the most powerful.

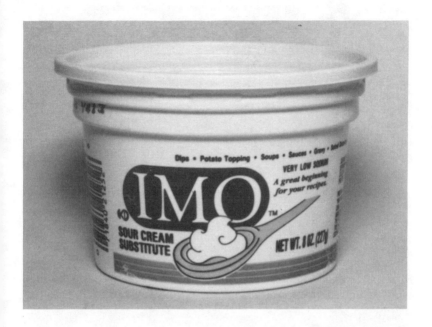

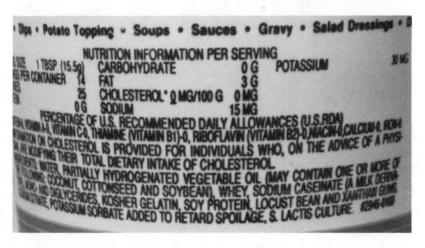

IMO™ is a sour cream substitute. It contains sodium caseinate, the milk protein, and will cause a reaction if you are sensitive to casein.

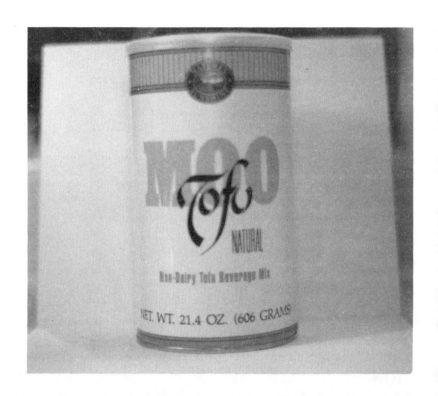

INGREDIENTS

Cereal solids (from corn), partially hydrogenated soy oil, dehydrated tofu, calcium carbonate, sodium caseinate, sea salt, fructose, natural flavors.

This product also claims to be non dairy, but contains sodium caseinate, a derivative of the milk protein. Even though this product is a supposed health supplement and is "Natural," it will cause problems for those who are allergic to casein.

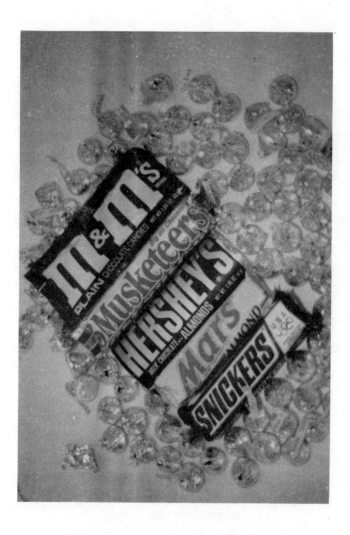

Chocolate is certainly the devil's food. It tastes great, it's addictive for some, and causes severe reactions in sensitive individuals. Almost all people who react to milk and dairy products also react to chocolate, only worse. It not only causes severe neck pain, back pain, and/or headaches in sensitive individuals, but can also cause irritability, depression, and anxiety.

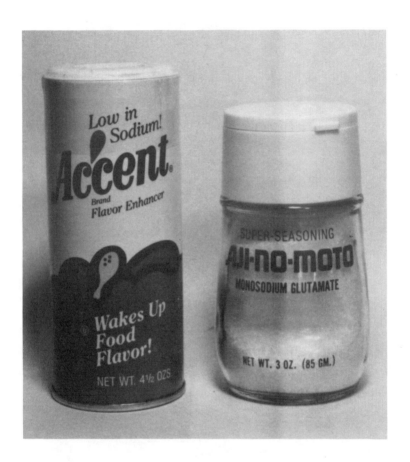

Monosodium Glutamate

These flavor enhancers, Accent and Aji-no-moto, are pure monosodium glutamate (MSG). Although pure MSG has no taste of its own, it enhances the flavor of any food to which it is added by stimulating the taste buds. Any food that boasts a "fuller" or "zesty" flavor should be suspected of containing MSG. Pure MSG can be found in almost any restaurant kitchen. If you eat out, *anywhere*, you are likely to be exposed to this powerful neuro-stimulator.

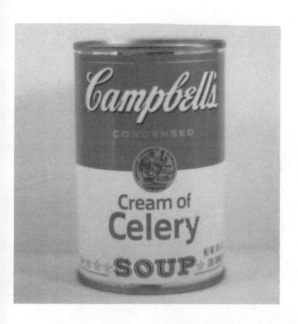

INGREDIENTS: WATER, CELERY, WHEAT FLOUR, VEGETABLE OIL (CORN, COTTONSEED OIL OR PARTIALLY HYDROGENATED SOYBEAN OIL), CREAM, SALT, CORNSTARCH, DRIED DAIRY BLEND (WHEY, CALCIUM CASEINATE), MARGARINE (PARTIALLY HYDROGENATED SOYBEAN OIL, WATER AND BETA CAROTENE FOR COLOR), WHEY, MONOSODIUM GLUTAMATE, SOY PROTEIN ISOLATE, NATURAL FLAVORING AND YEAST EXTRACT.

Soups and broths almost always contain MSG. Most Campbell's™ soups contain MSG. Here it is listed as monosodium glutamate and again as natural flavoring (may contain MSG). The only soup to trust is homemade—made by you, or someone you can trust who does not use MSG.

157

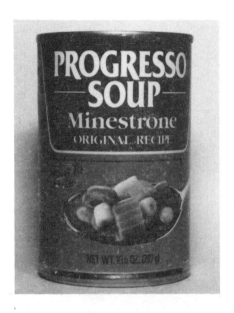

INGREDIENTS: WATER, RED KIDNEY BEANS, GREAT NORTHERN BEANS, LIMA BEANS, GREEN PEAS, CARROTS, CELERY, CABBAGE, GREEN BEANS, POTATOES, TOMATO PASTE, CHICK PEAS, ENRICHED MACARONI PRODUCT, SALT, SOYBEAN OIL, DEHYDRATED ONIONS, OLIVE OIL, GARLIC POWDER, SPICE, NATURAL FLAVOR.

Because of weak labelling laws, we have to wonder if this soup contains MSG. The last ingredient on this label is "Natural Flavors." MSG can be one of the ingredients in natural flavors. The law does not require the manufacturer to list MSG if it is included in the natural flavors.

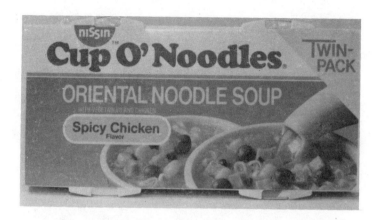

INGREDIENTS: ENRICHED WHEAT FLOUR (WHEAT FLOUR, NIACIN, REDUCED IRON, THIAMINE MONO-NITRATE, RIBOFLAVIN), PARTIALLY HYDROGENATED COTTONSEED OIL, DEHYDRATED VEGETABLES (CORN, CARROT, GREEN PEA, CHIVE), SALT, SOY SAUCE POWDER, FREEZE DRIED CHICKEN (CHICKEN MEAT, TEXTURED SOY FLOUR), DEXTROSE, MONOSODIUM GLUTAMATE, NATURAL FLAVORS, HYDROLYZED VEGETABLE PROTEINS, ONION POWDER, SPICES, GARLIC POWDER, VINEGAR POWDER, CHICKEN FAT, SHRIMP POWDER, CHICKEN POWDER, CITRIC ACID, POTASSIUM CARBONATE, SODIUM CARBONATE, TURMERIC AND CARROT OLEORESINS AS COLOR, DISODIUM GUANYLATE, DISODIUM INOSINATE, ARTIFICIAL FLAVORS, SODIUM ALGINATE, SUGAR, SODIUM TRIPOLYPHOSPHATE, TOCOPHEROLS AND SODIUM CITRATE.

Instant powdered soups like this one usually contain very high doses of MSG. Here we see it throughout the label as monosodium glutamate, natural flavors (may contain MSG), and hydrolyzed vegetable proteins (contains MSG). Lipton™, Top Ramen™, and many other manufacturers use high doses of MSG to enhance the flavor of their freezed and dried vegetables. Isn't it a shame that many doting mom's give their kids soup when they are sick or cold.

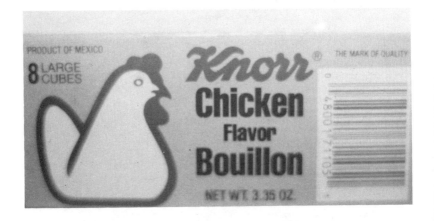

These bouillon cubes also contain a high dose of MSG. Here we see it listed as monosodium glutamate, hydrolyzed vegetable protein, yeast extract, natural flavors, and MSG is most likely in the broth.

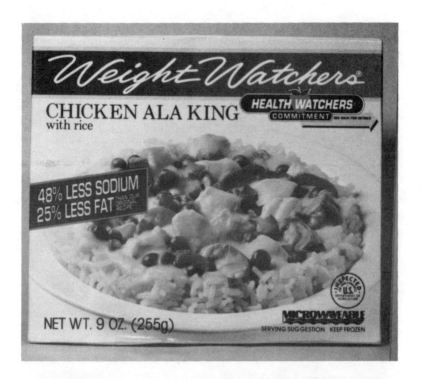

INGREDIENTS
RECONSTITUTED SKIM MILK, COOKED WHITE RICE, COOKED CHICKEN MEAT INCLUDING NATURAL CHICKEN JUICES, PEAS, MUSHROOMS, MODIFIED FOOD STARCH, RED PEPPERS, CELERY, CORN OIL, GREEN PEPPERS, FLOUR, SALT, HYDROLYZED VEGETABLE PROTEIN, MONOSODIUM GLUTAMATE, SUGAR, FLAVORINGS, DRIED WHEY, GRANULATED ONION, ONION POWDER, SPICE, TURMERIC, SHERRY WINE, SPICE EXTRACTIVES, CITRIC ACID.

Most instant TV dinners contain MSG. Many diet programs utilize these instant dinners that are loaded with MSG. This Weight Watcher's™ dinner advertises less sodium and less fat. But a closer look at the label reveals monosodium glutamate, hydrolyzed vegetable protein (contains MSG), and flavorings (may contain MSG). You may also take note of the first item on the label: milk.

161

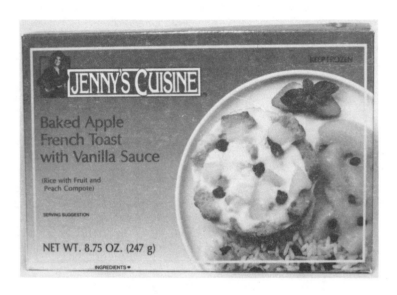

Jenny's Cuisine Salisbury Steak Champignon

(Salisbury Steak with Mushroom Sauce), Au Gratin Potatoes and Green Beans with Carrots in Sauce

INGREDIENTS: Cooked Beef, Water, Cooked Potatoes, Carrots, Green Beans, Onions, Cheddar Cheese, Bread Crumbs, Eggs, Mushrooms, White Wine, Margarine, Vegetable Oil, Demi Glace (Wheat Flour, Starch, Lactose, Dehydrated Onions, Salt, Tomato Starch, Hydrolyzed Plant Protein, Vegetable Oil, Yeast Extract, Beef Extract, Sugar, Caramel, Cornstarch, Wine Powder, Spices), Modified Food Starch, Tomato Paste, Nonfat Dry Milk, Salt, Flour, Natural Flavorings, Beef Flavor (Salt, Corn Syrup Solids, Beef Fat, Hydrolyzed Plant Protein, Celery and other Spices, Onion Powder, Starch, Beef Extract, Caramel Color, Garlic Powder, Spice Extractives of Pepper, Disodium Inosinate and Disodium Guanylate), Worcestershire Sauce, Spices, Chicken Flavor (Corn Syrup Solids, Salt, Chicken Fat, All Vegetable Shortening [Soybean, Cottonseed Oil], Onion Powder, Starch, Disodium Inosinate, Disodium Guanylate, Spice Extractives of Celery and Turmeric), Garlic, Parsley, Xanthan Gum, Annatto Color, Artificial Color (Contains FD&C Yellow #5).

PREPARED EXPRESSLY FOR
JENNY CRAIG, INC. · DEL MAR, CA 92014

Jenny Craig™ is another popular diet program that utilizes instant TV dinners. This offering of Jenny's Cuisine lists hydrolyzed plant protein in several places. Jenny Craig™ uses MSG.

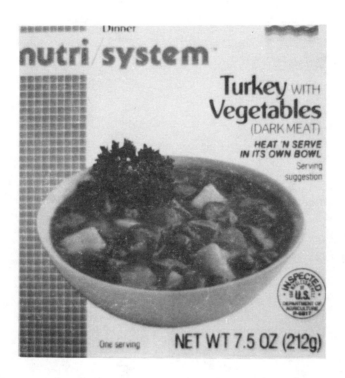

INGREDIENTS: CHICKEN BROTH, DARK TURKEY MEAT, RECONSTITUTED DEHYDROFROZEN POTATOES, WATER, ONIONS, CARROTS, NATURAL FLAVORING, PEAS, CELERY, MODIFIED FOOD STARCH, SOYBEAN OIL, WHEAT FLOUR, SUGAR, CORN FLOUR, SALT, DEHYDRATED BELL PEPPERS, DEHYDRATED CARROTS, FLAVORING.

Nutri/System™ is yet another popular diet program that relies on packaged frozen dinners. To provide a tasty product, they too use MSG. Here, the first item listed is chicken broth, undoubtedly containing MSG. "Natural flavoring" and "flavoring" also appear on this label and could contain MSG.

163

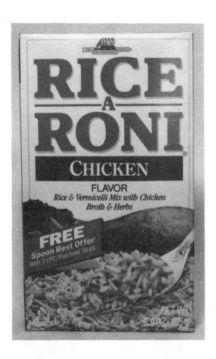

INGREDIENTS

ENRICHED RICE [RICE, NIACIN, IRON (FERRIC ORTHOPHOSPHATE, REDUCED IRON), THIAMINE MONONITRATE], ENRICHED VERMICELLI [FLOUR, NIACIN, IRON (FERROUS SULFATE), THIAMINE MONONITRATE, RIBOFLAVIN], SALT, FOOD STARCH-MODIFIED, SUGAR, YEAST EXTRACT,* CHICKEN FAT, NATURAL FLAVORS, ONIONS,* MONOSODIUM GLUTAMATE, CHICKEN BROTH,* CHICKEN,* PARSLEY,* YEAST,* SOY FLOUR, GARLIC,* SPICE, PARTIALLY HYDROGENATED VEGETABLE OIL (SOYBEAN AND/OR COTTONSEED), DISODIUM INOSINATE, DISODIUM GUANYLATE.
*DRIED

Brown rice and white rice are just too plain. So this product is spiced up. When a packaged food mentions the word "flavor" in prominence, suspect MSG. This label lists monosodium glutamate, and chicken broth, which contains MSG.

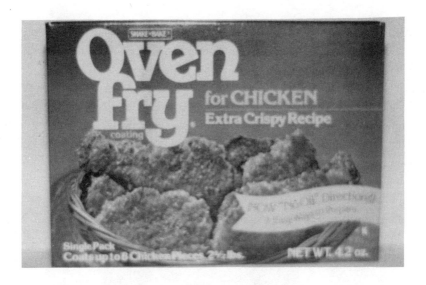

Most breadings on meats and deep fried vegetables are intended to add crunchiness and flavor. This Shake 'n Bake™ chicken
breading contains monosodium glutamate and hydrolyzed vegetable protein (contains MSG). "Natural Flavorings" also appears
on the label and may contain MSG as well.

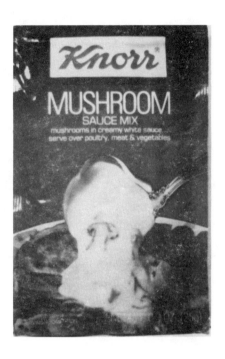

INGREDIENTS: WHEAT FLOUR, DEHYDRATED MUSHROOMS, PARTIALLY HYDROGENATED PEANUT OIL, HYDROLYZED VEGETABLE PROTEIN, NON-FAT DRY MILK, SALT, DEHYDRATED ONIONS, YEAST EXTRACT, STARCH, NATURAL FLAVORS, SOUP STOCK, MODIFIED FOOD STARCH, PAPRIKA, TURMERIC.

Many sauce mixes, or flavor packets contain MSG. This product contains hydrolyzed vegetable protein (contains MSG) and yeast extract. "Natural flavors" and "soup stock" are also listed and most likely contain MSG.

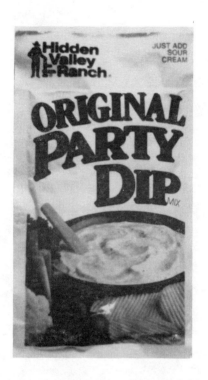

INGREDIENTS: MALTODEXTRIN, SALT, MONO-SODIUM GLUTAMATE, DEHYDRATED ONION, DEHYDRATED GARLIC, DEHYDRATED PARS-LEY, CARRAGEENAN, SPICE, CALCIUM STEARATE, AND SOYBEAN OIL. SODIUM CON-TENT PER TABLESPOON SERVING: 115MG AS PACKAGED AND 120MG AS PREPARED. LOW SODIUM PRODUCT.

This party dip lists monosodium glutamate as the third ingred-ient. Mixing the contents of the packet with sour cream could lead to a powerful reaction in any person who is sensitive to dairy products and/or MSG.

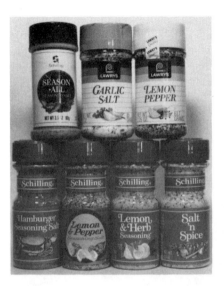

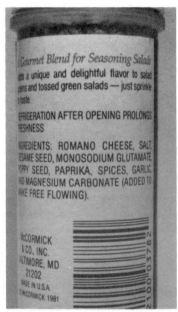

Gourmet Blend for Seasoning Salads

adds a unique and delightful flavor to salad greens and tossed green salads — just sprinkle to taste.

REFRIGERATION AFTER OPENING PROLONGS FRESHNESS

INGREDIENTS: ROMANO CHEESE, SALT, SESAME SEED, MONOSODIUM GLUTAMATE, POPPY SEED, PAPRIKA, SPICES, GARLIC AND MAGNESIUM CARBONATE (ADDED TO MAKE FREE FLOWING).

McCORMICK
& CO. INC.
BALTIMORE, MD
21202
MADE IN U.S.A.
© McCORMICK 1981

CONTAINS: BLACK PEPPER, SALT, MODIFIED FOOD STARCH, CITRIC ACID, LEMON PEEL, SUGAR, MONOSODIUM GLUTAMATE (FOR FULLER FLAVOR), GARLIC, ONION, NATURAL FLAVOR AND RIBOFLAVIN (FOR COLOR).   MADE IN U.S.A.

Many spices contain mixtures of herbs and spices and other flavor enhancers. All of the spices pictured here contain monosodium glutamate and/or natural flavorings. Many people assume that spices are harmless, however, many of them contain MSG. Lawry's™ Seasoning Salt is not pictured here, but contains MSG in the large size, but claims there is no MSG in the smaller sizes. Mrs. Dash™ contains natural flavors that may include MSG.

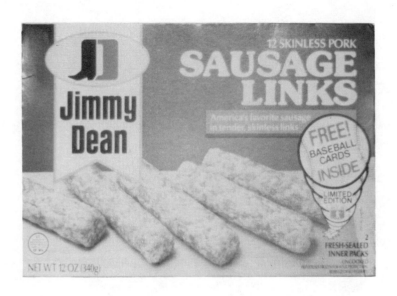

INGREDIENTS: PORK,
WATER, SALT, SPICES,
SUGAR, MONOSODIUM
GLUTAMATE.
DIST. BY JIMMY DEAN FOODS
CORDOVA, TN 38018

Many packaged meats contain MSG. These Jimmy Dean™ Sausage Links list monosodium glutamate on the label. In fact, most Jimmy Dean™ products use MSG.

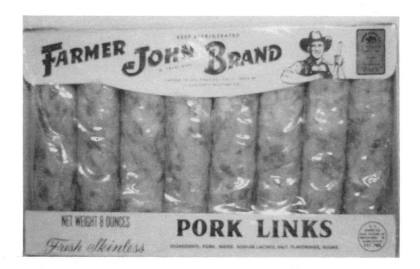

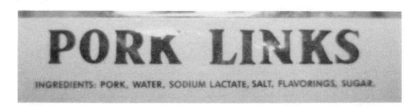

These Farmer John™ Pork Links do not list monosodium glutamate on the label. However, "flavorings" could, and most likely
does contain MSG. When "flavorings" or "natural flavorings"
appears on the label of a packaged meat, that product most
likely contains MSG. It's a shame we have to wonder. In fact, it's
a crime. Hopefully, labelling laws will change.

170

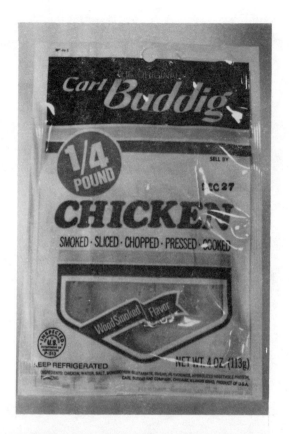

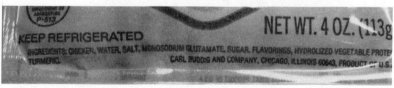

Many packaged lunch meats contain MSG. This particular brand lists monosodium glutamate as one of the ingredients. Other brands will not mention MSG, but will list "flavorings" or "natural flavorings." According to current law, it is legal for these food manufacturers to include MSG in flavorings and not mention it. My advice is: Don't wonder. If the label is not clear, don't buy it.

171

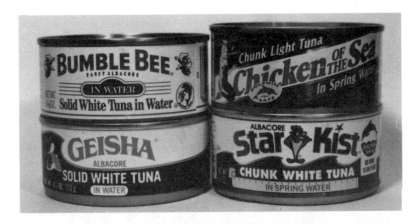

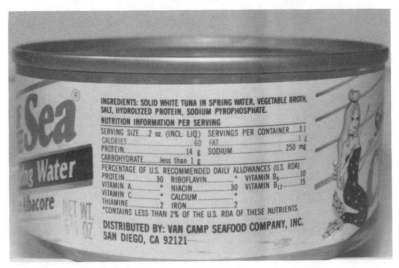

Most people are not aware that most tuna fish contains MSG. Many people I talk to believe they are making the healthy choice by buying tuna that is packed in water. Many of them believe that white tuna, or albacore is the best. Most people are not aware that tuna fish cans are labelled. Check it out sometime. All of the cans pictured here contain MSG. This Chicken of the Sea™ Solid White tuna in water is not just tuna and water. It also contains vegetable broth, which most likely contains MSG. Hydrolyzed vegetable protein contains MSG and is in this can of tuna.

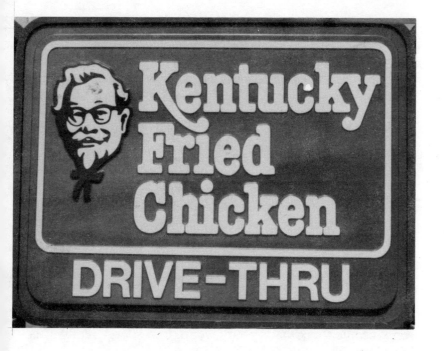

Most restaurants use MSG. Chinese restaurants are famous for their heavy use of MSG. But fast food restaurants and greasy spoons and even fancy restaurants use MSG. Many restaurants soak their salads in MSG. Most restaurants put MSG in their soups. Many sauces and spices at your favorite restaurants are spiked with MSG.

Guess what one of Colonel Sander's™ secret herbs and spices is? MSG.

173

4

The Symptoms

Because allergy is a systemic disorder, any part of the system can be involved, and virtually any symptom can occur. In Dr. Mandell's book, *Dr. Mandell's Five Day Allergy Relief System,* he tests patients with suspected allergens, usually foods, after five days of fasting. He watches for reactions after exposure to each suspected allergen. Now, if a patient's main complaint is headaches, and he or she reports that they got one after being challenged with, oh, let's say milk, that's a pretty subjective test. Maybe the patient lied. Maybe he or she succumbed to the power of suggestion.

To get a more objective result, Dr. Mandell took a handwriting sample after each challenge. Variations are noted. Now, some people think that's pretty weird. Can allergy really affect handwriting?

Yes. Handwriting is just a very finely tuned motor skill controlled by the nervous system. Most allergens have some effect on the nervous system, and any effect will become evident when the fine motor skill of handwriting is altered. If you look on page 184 of his book, you will see a sampling of handwriting reactions to food and mold challenges. This particular patient, a young girl, reversed letters in her name, and omitted others, after exposure to milk. Dr. Mandell has seen it. Dr.

174

Frank Oski has seen it. Many others have seen that milk and dairy products are the number one food allergy in children and the cause of many childhood problems, including learning disorders.

What are we doing to our kids? Many school lunches come with milk as the only beverage choice unless the child has a note from a doctor. We ought to print up a few million notes. I recently spoke with a special education teacher who saw a child have epileptic attacks after eating hot dogs at school. Hot dogs at school! He and the mother saw this several times. Baby food manufacturers stopped using MSG years ago, voluntarily, but schools still feed it to older kids. Does that make sense?

People don't consult me for learning disorders. I just see them along the way. I'm a chiropractor, so people consult me for neck pain, back pain, and headaches, usually. I have seen certain symptoms over and over again that are classically caused by allergy to casein. Casein is the main cause of neck pain, back pain, and headaches, but all these symptoms can be caused by other allergens. These symptoms are many times aggravated by other factors, or stressors, like trauma, or stress, or cold weather. But despite what other doctors will tell you, the main cause is the allergen. The other stressors will produce symptoms, in almost every case, **only** in the presence of the allergen, usually casein. Many arthritics tell me their joints are aggravated by cold, damp weather. And they are. So these people are flocking to Palm Springs and to the desert where I live. They have manipulated their environments to remove a stressor. However, in almost every case, these people will tolerate cold, damp weather when the chemical stressor, the allergen, or allergens, are eliminated.

The symptoms I see in my practice involve spinal pain and/or headaches. Although I see specific symptoms repeatedly, and relate these symptoms to patients looking for a causal connection, lack of these symptoms, or different combinations of symptoms, do not preclude allergy as a cause. Some patients listen intently to specific symptoms common in the milk connection, leaning forward, analyzing every word, then suddenly sigh and say, "Nope! That's not me. Those aren't my symptoms."

Again, symptoms due to allergy are caused by the allergen as it circulates through the blood. The symptoms can be anything and occur anywhere. The symptoms, or pain, often move, or seems to migrate. Moving pain, especially leg or arm numbness or pain that switches from right to left, is a definite indicator that a chemical cause should be considered over a mechanical cause.

Neck and Upper Back Symptoms

The most common musculoskeletal complaint due to a reaction to casein is neck stiffness, often radiating across the shoulders. Generalized stiffness throughout the spine, in fact, is common, affecting the right and left sides. Many of these patients are constantly rubbing their necks, rotating their heads, trying to get some flexibility. Many of them will need nightly neck rubs from their spouses. The spouses have noticed "knots" in the shoulders.

Equally common, perhaps even more common, is upper back and neck pain that occurs on one side. In fact, one sided symptoms are very common in allergy. Ear infections usually occur on only one side. Many patients experience all of their symptoms on one side with the head and back, arm and leg of the right or left side being involved.

This neck and upper back pain usually starts as a knot, or burning pain between the shoulder blades, usually off to one side of the spine under the scapula (the wing bone on the back). Many people with this complaint describe the sensation as a pressure, or "it feels like I'm laying on a golf ball." The pain radiates up to the shoulder and continues up into the neck on the same side, often radiating over the ear into the temple and into the eye, usually just the one. (See cover.) This half-head headache is the classic allergy headache. A common description is "It feels like my eye is going to explode."

This one sided shoulder blade pain that radiates into the neck usually occurs on one side, usually the same side. But many patients notice that once in a while it "shifts" to the other side. Sometimes it will radiate into the arm and/or hand on the same side, as numbness, tingling, muscle weakness, or pain.

The most classic musculoskeletal symptom of milk allergy is cracking and popping, or grinding and crunching noises in the neck. Doctors and medical students call this crepitus, a great word to know to impress your friends. But the significance of crepitus was never pointed out to me in school. Just something to notice and name. Many patients notice these noises in their necks, and many times in other joints throughout their bodies. Some of these patients claim to get relief by "cracking" their necks. Many of them are proud to report to me that they are able to "adjust" their own necks. Crepitus is common also in the knees and ankles.

Crepitus is not present in every case of milk allergy. In my experience, crepitus is present in 75% of cases where symptoms are due to milk allergy. But, crepitus will disappear in 99% of cases when casein is totally eliminated from the diet. **After casein is totally eliminated, crepitus will disappear, usually in two to three weeks.** I have seen that fail only a handful of times. So I use crepitus as a strong indicator of the presence of casein in the diet.

When a patient fails to respond after a reasonable time, or has a recurrence of symptoms, I will begin by asking questions about the diet, looking for casein. If the patient denies using dairy foods, I ask them if they are experiencing cracking and popping in the neck. A "yes" answer calls for more aggressive questioning to find the casein in the diet. It could be hidden, or not obvious to the patient. Many times a patient will start on a diet that consists of a protein shake once or several times a day. Most of these shakes are mixed with milk, but, for some reason, this milk use escapes the awareness of some people, even ones who are sincerely trying to avoid milk. Still others will mix the powder with a soy milk in an attempt to avoid casein.

But most of these powders already contain milk, or sodium caseinate.

Sometimes patients lie. It's difficult, and certainly not to my liking, to suspect that a patient is lying. But it happens, and must be considered. The most dishonest, or difficult group to manage (in my experience) are in the age range of 15 years of age to the early twenties. Most of these kids are beyond parental control. They don't pay attention to what they eat. It's a low priority. They eat a lot of fast food, and besides, they're in the prime of their lives — not a time to be giving up the goodies that all their friends are eating in front of their faces.

I once attempted to manage the diet of a 19 year old male (man or boy, who knows?). He was, and is, such a nice guy. He had the exuberance of youth, and a great smile. He weighed 224 pounds. When I suggested a diet change for him, he got enthusiastic. He jumped on the scale, seemed highly motivated by my suggestions, and began his strict new diet. Each time he came into the office for treatment, I would ask him what he had eaten since the last visit. In the beginning, I would catch dairy "slip ups" after he experienced recurrences of symptoms (low back pain, in his case). After I pointed out the milk connection to him several times, he became more steadfast in his diet. He was really involved now. He told me so. But once, after I hadn't seen him for a full week, I asked him how he was eating.

"I'm on a strict diet now. I haven't eaten all week."

"Nothing?" I asked.

"Nope. Just water. Well, I think I had a salad two days ago."

Sounds fishy, huh? I put him on the scale and he had gained seven pounds in that one week alone! He was shocked. He couldn't believe it. He insisted on sticking to his story.

I said, "Sure Freddy."

He gave me a sly smile as he walked out the door.

So I ask about crepitus. If they have it, they're most likely having casein.

Tingling and numbness in the hands and/or feet (parasthesias) is a very common symptom of milk allergy. It usually occurs in both hands, sometimes one worse than the other, and sometimes only in one hand. The common medical diagnosis for this symptom is carpal tunnel syndrome. (There's that word "syndrome" again, a strong indicator that the cause is unknown.)

I think carpal tunnel syndrome is a sad diagnosis. The carpal tunnel is in the wrist. It is a passageway made up of bone and soft tissue that encases some blood vessels and the median and radial nerves supplying the hand. The typical medical explanation of the disorder is that scar tissue in the tunnel has interfered with the nerves. This scar tissue has developed from overuse of the hands, like typing, or using a jackhammer, or bicycling, or gymnastics. But, as most doctors know, carpal tunnel syndrome occurs in many, many people who have no such history. Carpal tunnel surgery is performed, sadly enough, very often. It is designed, I guess, to clear out the canal. Results are very poor. Extremely poor. This surgery usually creates more scar tissue than it eliminates. The doctors are slashing wrists and getting paid for it. Poor results don't slow them down. In fact, poor results to some doctors mean "do it again."

Tingling and numbness in the hands, or pain, or cold hands is almost always allergy, usually to casein. Even when the patient has a physical history that would justify a mechanical cause, a chemical change, usually eliminating casein, will solve the problem. Surgery is unnecessary.

Sometimes this tingling and numbness will occur in the feet, one or both. Whether in the hands, or in the feet, many times only one side will be involved, but sometimes the symptoms will switch to the other side. Any time pain or numbness radiates into the extremities (called radicular pain, or parasthesias), most conventional medics assume a physical irritation of the nerve has occurred. The nerves that supply the upper extremities exit the spinal column in the cervical spine, the neck. Many athletes have experienced a "zinger" down the arm after getting their necks twisted, or after jamming their heads into another athlete. This is a graphic example of a physical irritation of a nerve root (in the neck), causing radicular symptoms (pain or numbness in the hands or arms). Usually symptoms in these instances occur on one side only. If the injury causes permanent damage, the symptoms will persist, or recur, always on the same side.

Most of us have experienced the sleeping leg that has been crossed too long. The nerve is physically irritated at the hip or behind the knee, causing radicular symptoms.

Many surgeries are performed with the aid of a "saddle block." In these surgeries, the spinal cord is injected with an anesthetic to deaden the sensory nerves to the pelvis, so pelvic surgery can be performed. When surgery is to be performed on a knee, the anesthesia is injected into the lower back, where the nerve roots exit to supply the lower extremities. When the patient is rolled onto his side, with the right side down, the anesthesia flows onto the right nerve roots, and the right leg goes numb. This is an example of a chemical irritant.

Other examples of chemical irritants causing parasthesias, or radicultitis, or numbness and tingling in the extremities, are listed in the Physician's Desk Reference (PDR). Look under the section headed "Adverse Reactions" and you will notice that many drugs cause these symptoms inadvertently. I have had patients consult me for these parasthesias that were merely side effects of medications they were taking. My treatment consisted of giving them a photocopy of the page from the PDR that dealt with their particular drug. Then I instructed the patient to consult the doctor who prescribed the drug. Good luck.

So, even though medical doctors are aware that nerves can be irritated both physically and chemically, they almost always consider only the physical irritation, even when there is no history of physical trauma. In my experience, chemical irritation is almost always a factor, even when there is also a physical irritation. In most cases of tingling and numbness in the extremities, the irritation is chemical, usually allergy to casein.

Headaches

Headaches are the bane of our modern, stressful, technological society. Headaches can be caused by brain tumors and concussions. Headaches can be caused by polyps in the brain. Headaches can be caused by medication. These causes are the culprit in headache sufferers in less than one percent of headaches. But the medical profession insists on focusing on these causes. They order CT scans, x-rays, blood tests, eye tests. When the results are negative, as they almost always are, they order more tests. While this pointless medical charade goes on and on and on, the patient is bombarded with different medications, or shots of demerol if the pain is severe enough.

To consult a medical doctor for headaches is pointless, unless he or she practices bio ecology. They have only one treatment for headaches, and that is medication. Oh, they have a lot of different ones, but the only difference is the side effects. Many patients report to me that, after consulting lots of doctors, they finally found one who discovered what their problem was: Migraines.

That is the most dead-end diagnosis I have ever heard. Migraine is no diagnosis at all. It just means that you have severe headaches. Oh, they get more technical than that. It's vascular, and you can feel it coming on. Most headache sufferers can figure that much out without a doctor. Migraine is a dead-end diagnosis because that's where the case usually ends — with the diagnosis. No hope is offered, and sufferers assume, and are often told, that there is no cure but to take medication. They're often told it's hereditary or stress.

Sometimes extensive testing will end in a diagnosis of "cluster headaches." These come on for several hours or days, then go away, and are relieved sometimes by coffee. Again, that is not a diagnosis. That is only a description of the headaches. Putting a name to symptoms and charging money for it is not health care. But I guess it's what some people are used to.

No Milk

I always ask patients if they get headaches. Some of the answers amaze me, like "Oh just normal headaches, not often."

"Not often" is an answer that always calls for clarification. I've heard "Only once a day" several times! Some people think headaches once a week, or once a month are normal. **No headache is normal.** Some people think they deserve headaches.

A very common answer I get when I ask if a patient gets headaches is, "No. Just sinus." Like what they think is a sinus headache is normal. Sinus headaches are not normal. Cluster headaches are not normal. Migraines are not normal. Headaches once in a while are not normal.

People like to go to great lengths to describe their headaches to me. They get really descriptive. They know their headaches. I've heard many, many, many very interesting descriptions. I listen and I take notes because I find it fascinating and I like to see similar stories. I listen because I always feel I can learn something.

Once a patient described her headaches to me, using words like "itching," "burning," "ants," and "knives." She went on and on in great detail. When she was done, I looked up from my notes and she was staring at me with her mouth open.

"What's wrong?" I asked.

"You're the first doctor that didn't tell me I was crazy!"

You see, headaches come in all sizes and shapes, and it is interesting to hear the different descriptions, but actually unnecessary. But after listening to many descriptions, the most common headache is the half-head headache that begins at the base of the skull, behind the ear on one side. From there, it radiates over the ear to the temple and into the eye. Another classic description is the headache that happens around the eyes. Many times, the eyes are sensitive to light. This occurs so often that I always include it in my verbal symptom survey. Many times the pressure in the eye causes the affected eye to appear bloodshot.

However, the only really important information is that the patient does get headaches. From there, I need only to know how often, when, and how long do they last. A headache is only an indication that something is wrong, something is circulating in the blood. We need to know when it occurs so we can find out what's in the blood at the time. What's in the diet (or the air) is what's in the blood.

Solving headaches is more investigative work than it is doctoring.

Headaches are always reactions to something, almost always allergy, almost always food. I tell patients that all headaches are caused by something that was breathed in or eaten. To solve headaches, we need to know when they happen, and what happened to cause them. If a patient is getting headaches all the time, or every day, I look first for a food that is a regular part of the diet. If headaches occur only once in a while, we need to isolate one, then establish the dietary events that preceded the headache. We will not be looking for a food that is eaten every day, in this case, otherwise the headaches would occur more often. Most headaches occur in the frequency range of two or three a week.

Many women who suffer with premenstrual syndrome (PMS), experience headaches along with all the other misery of the syndrome. These headaches occur only once a month with the menstrual cycle. The assumption by many, is that these headaches can only be avoided by ripping out the uterus, a hysterectomy, or by taking the pill, or hormones. But a thorough history will usually reveal that cravings for certain foods, usually chocolate, are part of the PMS experience. Chocolate, as I have discussed, is the most powerful cause of back pain and headaches. Chocolate also causes mood changes in some people, usually irritability, depression, and anxiety. Sounds like PMS, huh? Most of the PMS symptoms, including headaches, can be controlled, or eliminated by dietary manipulation. I advise the elimination of dairy products, including chocolate, also caffeine, sugar, salt, nicotine, and all chemicals. It seems the system is more sensitive to irritants, allergens, and poisons during the menstrual cycle.

No Milk

Some women claim their husbands or mates suffer from PMS. They see mood changes, short tempers, depression, etc. in their men. The most common causes are chocolate, or drugs, many times cocaine or methamphetamine (speed). Allergens can also cause these mood swings. I have seen adults and children who react with rage to dairy products.

The most common cause of headaches is casein. In my practice, I have seen that **95% of all headaches are caused by casein.** Almost all others are caused by MSG. Any headache can be solved if the patient is cooperative. A thorough history, a diet diary, and persistence will solve nearly every headache case. I have not seen one headache in the last four years that was not dietary in origin. In the next chapter I have included several headache cases that go beyond the milk connection.**As a basic rule, headaches are caused by exposure to an allergen or poison, or withdrawal from one.** Remember that headache is one of the classic withdrawal symptoms.

So many times, when a patient complains of symptoms, like headaches, mood swings, etc., and the doctors can't figure out why, they blame the symptoms on stress. **Stress,** like cold weather, is just another factor that can stress the system and contribute to symptoms. But stress affects different people in different ways. Some people get headaches, some get tightness in the neck and shoulders, some get upset stomachs, some sweat, some cry, some shake, and on and on. That's because stress will affect a person where there is a pre-existing weakness. **Stress will not cause physical symptoms when the cause of the pre-existing weakness is eliminated.** For example, a difficult discussion with your signifigant-other will have a different outcome after a pot of coffee or a keg of beer.

The main cause is almost never stress. So, before you get divorced, or quit your job, or sell your kids, consider your diet.

Low Back Pain

The most common work related injury is to the low back. In the state of California, employers are responsible for medical treatment for low back injuries that happen to employees while they are on the job. Usually , the only relationship between the back pain and the job is time and location. The cause is usually casein, many times chocolate and/or ice cream, inflaming the joints and muscles, aggravated by some activity that happens to take place at work. The employer is suddenly responsible for the employees dietary habits because no one has made the connection.

I describe that scenario, not to ruffle feathers, but because it happens that way so often.

But to move on, the most common low back complaint due to milk allergy is stiffness in the muscles of the low back, usually worse in the morning. Many patients complain that they have difficulty lifting their legs to put their shoes on. Some people experience leg pain or numbness, in one or both legs. Sometimes the legs feel weak. Leg cramping due to casein is very common. **In fact, the most common cause of leg cramping is casein.** Many people recognize the common name, **sciatica**, inflammation of the sciatic nerve in the leg. The most common medical explanation of leg pain is that it is caused by a pinched nerve in the low back, usually due to a disc protrusion, or herniation, or arthritic spurs. The assumption is that low back pain is due to physical trauma, and certainly a physical act set off the pain, so the doctors look for a physical explanation for the symptoms. An x-ray picture, or a CT scan, will sometimes show some degenerative changes, or calcium deposits, or a bulging disc or two. In these cases, the doctors usually recommend surgery or medication. The assumption is that physical abnormalities visible in an x-ray picture of the low back are the cause of the symptoms.

However, many studies have been conducted where x-rays and CT scans were taken of patients who had no complaints of low back pain, and guess what? Lots of these asymptomatic patients had bulging discs and degenerative changes in the low back. In other studies, patients who experienced low back pain received CT scans that revealed bulging discs. After successful treatment with physical therapy, or chiropractic care, the symptoms went away. A new CT scan of the now pain-free low back showed the same bulging discs.

Again, most low back pain is due to a chemical irritant, an allergen, usually casein.

Joint Pain

It seems that musculoskeletal pain due to allergy to casein is due to inflammation of the joints. It follows logically, that any joint can be involved. *Arthritis* is the Greek and Latin translation of *inflammation of the joints*. *Rheumatoid arthritis* is a more specific diagnosis that is translated into conventional medicine as *no hope*. Arthritis, or inflammation of the joints, can be due to wear and tear on joints, like the knees of football players. But when all of the joints are involved, the cause is not physical, but chemical. In systemic arthritis, like rheumatoid, the cause is coursing through the blood, and it got there from the diet. It's usually casein, but other allergens can cause the same symptoms. Conventional doctors prefer to consider the cause of arthritis to be hereditary, or unknown.

I once saw a 65 year old man, Bob, who complained of neck stiffness and headaches. I instructed him to eliminate all milk and dairy products. He came in only one time. He lived in a small town about 25 miles from my office. Several months later, I began seeing an influx of patients from that town, all referred by Bob. One of these referrals was another retired gentleman who was good friends with Bob. He told me that Bob had eliminated milk products successfully and was no longer experiencing his neck pain and headaches. But more amazingly, this man reported, Bob lived to play golf, and he was about to give up the game because his hands were always so stiff and sore, he could barely grip the clubs. Since quitting dairy products, his hands were also now pain free.

Joy, a 42 year old woman consulted me for headaches. After eliminating dairy products, her headaches were gone. She noticed also that her painful knees, diagnosed as arthritic, were pain free since milk had been eliminated. Once, after drinking a glass of milk, her knees swelled within 20 minutes.

Painful, swollen, or stiff joints — one, or several, or all — are common complaints of allergy to casein. Stiffness in the hands is a common complaint. Sometimes, only one joint is involved.

It must be understood that other allergens can cause the same symptoms. Corn, wheat, and soy have also been known to cause arthritic changes in sensitive individuals.

Other Symptoms

Decreased energy, or fatigue, is a common symptom of food allergy. Many people have experienced sudden drowsiness after a meal. Many women, who have suffered with chronic fatigue for years, and have consulted conventional doctors, are taking thyroid medication. Almost all of these patients would have gotten relief with dietary manipulation, usually by avoiding milk and dairy products.

Many times, allergens, especially casein, will have an effect on the vascular system. One of the classic symptoms of milk allergy is that the eyes are sensitive to light. The blood vessels in the back of the eyeball, on the retina, are the smallest, most fragile blood vessels in the body. Doctors examine these blood vessels in a physical exam because, many times, the first signs of high blood pressure, or diabetes, or other systemic diseases that affect the vascular system, will affect these small blood vessels first. Allergens, like casein, that affect blood vessels, will often cause the eyes to be sensitive to light. Sometimes patients describe a feeling of pressure behind the eyes.

Dizziness is one of the more common symptoms of allergy to casein. Some people believe it's normal to get dizzy when getting up, or bending over. When headaches and dizziness occur together, conventional doctors usually blame blood pressure. Again, high blood pressure is another common symptom of food allergy, not the cause of symptoms.

Allergens that affect the blood vessels can cause symptoms in other organs. **In patients where allergy to casein has been established, I have seen a high incidence of endometriosis (inflammation of the uterus), and varicose veins.**

The most common cause of **sinus congestion** and runny noses is milk and dairy products. Many people who suffer with sinus problems blame them on dusts and pollens, or the wind. Certainly these contribute to and aggravate sinus problems. However, in many cases, dust and pollen and wind will not cause sinus problems when milk products are eliminated from the diet.

The skin can also be affected. Allergy to casein can cause **eczema** in children, **rashes**, and **cysts**. There is also a high incidence of **ovarian cysts** in women with allergy to casein. Allergy to dairy products manifests itself in teenagers as **acne**.

Moods and personalities are often affected by allergens and poisons. We know that people who are under the influence of alcohol or PCP often act inappropriately. Many of us have experienced the irritability that accompanies the jitters after too much coffee.

Depression and listlessness and a quick-to-temper attitude are often, in fact **usually** reactions of the central nervous system to allergens or poisons. Many of us have experienced those days when we feel grouchy, or out of sorts for no apparent reason.

Certainly many people experience mood swings because of their condition, or the way their day is going, or because of a traumatic past, etc. But many times we all assume that these upsets are the only causes of emotional disturbances or mood swings. This is not true. The ebb and flow of a person's moods and/or psychological state is more affected by chemical agents than by that person's perception of surrounding events.

But people who seek professional help for depression, or mood swings, or anger tendencies usually receive counseling, a closer look at their pasts, their relationships with their mothers and fathers, and the other emotional stresses in their lives. To compliment the counseling, they get to take some drugs: uppers if they're too low, downers if they're too high, stabilizers if they're up and down, sedatives if they're not sedate enough for society, experimental drugs if the others don't work.

Stress as a health risk is getting a lot of press lately. I agree that we should all give up our fast paced jobs and leave the cities and go live on farms, but who would manufacture our supplies and hook up our cable? Besides, a lot of people handle a lot of stress, often times much more stress than those that are complaining, and it doesn't make them sick or unhappy.

Treatment programs designed to reduce stress, perceptually and chemically, should be a last resort, not a big industry. I believe that all people are basically good, level-headed, loving, caring individuals. Some people have been raised in bad environments and believe that yelling and screaming and beating and crying are normal. They were taught that by people who were taught that because they didn't know any other way. But the vast majority of us can handle stressful situations without coming unglued, or depressed, or sick, or disabled. As long as we are not under the influence of alcohol, or caffeine, or drugs, or allergens or poisons that cause irritation of the nervous system and thereby producing mood swings and the apparent inability to handle stress.

To be totally at peace can only be attained by avoiding stimulants and depressants and allergens and poisons — in short, chemicals that alter the harmonious functioning of the nervous system. Do that first, before you quit your job or send your wife or husband or kids packing.

These are some of the symptoms I have seen over and over again due to allergy to casein. I'm sure there are many, many more that will become apparent to me, and those who pay attention, as time goes by. The point is, an allergen, or poison, circulating through the blood can affect any tissue that it contacts, and can therefor cause any symptom.

No Milk

I took many classes in diagnosis in school. Most of them involved memorizing lists of signs and symptoms that were classic for each disease or disorder. When a test question asked for a description of a specific disease, it was fairly easy (after lots of study) to regurgitate the classic list of signs and symptoms. Conversely, a classic list of signs and symptoms was easy to recognize and name with the appropriate disease. But one time I took a test that didn't seem to make sense. On this test, a list of symptoms to be named would appear incomplete. Or the list would include classic symptoms of several diseases. I was confused. The whole class was confused. We thought the teacher must have been drinking when making up the test. When we pointed out the apparent errors to the teacher, she just smiled and said, "Welcome to clinical diagnosis. Patients rarely come in to a clinic with 'classic symptoms.' And," she pointed out, "they will never hand you a nice, neat list of their complaints."

This is true. I have seen many, many different combinations of the "classic" symptoms. This chapter has been a reporting of the "classic" symptoms I have seen caused by allergy to casein. But remember, any symptom can be caused by allergy, and any allergen can cause any symptom.

We need to study other diseases and symptoms and establish dietary connections. Doctors collect all sorts of data on cancer patients that have to do with race, sex, age, where they live, etc. They use these statistics to help you calculate your risk of getting certain kinds of cancer. How about collecting dietary habits of cancer patients, then stick that information in a computer? I think we would learn a lot.

I have my suspicions. Exposure to allergens causes stress to the system. Continued exposure causes continued stress and continued tissue breakdown. I have seen a progression of symptoms in people who continue to expose themselves to allergens. Their symptoms go from bad to worse. Ear infections become headaches that become back aches that become ulcers. Then the gall bladder comes out. Then a hysterectomy. Then thyroid medication. Then bypass surgery. What's next?

Does leukemia occur in people who don't drink cow's milk? How many heart attacks are preceded by the ingestion of MSG? Has anyone asked these questions?

I wonder.

5

The Stories

Nick, a 42 year old Greek immigrant, complained of intense headaches that he had been experiencing for nearly two years. He had these headaches every day. They started nearly two years ago for no apparent reason. He had had no auto accidents, or falls, and could remember nothing in the way of trauma that could have brought them on. In fact, he had made absolutely no changes in any aspect of his life. His diet was the same. He had the same job, the same wife, lived in the same house, etc. The pain started on the right side of his neck behind his right ear, then radiated over his right ear to his right eye. He felt an intense pressure in his right eye. He said it felt like it was going to explode. Bright light bothered him. He had been to every specialist he could think of, his general physician, neurologists, orthopedists, and internists. He had had CT scans, x-rays, and blood tests. Nothing showed up on any of the tests. The doctors were trying to solve his problem by trying different medications. He was now on ibuprofen and codeine. They were not helping. The doctors told him that he must reduce stress in his life. Right. He had virtually given up. A friend dragged him into my office against his will. He told me so. He said he didn't want to be there. He was tired of doctors. The history revealed that he was a heavy milk drinker. I treated him three times and took him off all dairy products. His headaches were gone in four days.

Diane, a 21 year old female college student came into my office complaining of a sharp pain and feeling of pressure between her spine and scapula (wing bone on the back). When she would lie on her back, it felt as though a fist, or a golf ball was under her in this spot. The pain radiated to her neck and head on the right side. This pain syndrome occurred almost always on the right, but every once in a while it switched to the left. She had been going to M.D.'s for two years who were specialists in **myofascial pain syndrome**, the common medical diagnosis for these symptoms. She was getting treatment three times a week. Treatment included spraying fluoro-methane (Spray and Stretch™) on the area of pain while her head was pulled down and forward to stretch the involved muscles. This was followed by injections of xylocaine into the trigger points, the main areas of pain. After two years of treatment, she was still suffering from the same symptoms. When she eliminated milk and dairy products from her diet, her pain stopped.

A 45 year old female, Tootsie, complained of neck pain and headaches similar to the ones described above. They would come on once or twice a month for no apparent reason. They mainly occurred on the right, but sometimes would happen on the left. She was in great shape from doing aerobics, but had quit because she feared they were causing her problem. She had been going to chiropractors for years. She came in when I was first discovering the milk connection. At first I didn't make the connection, and when I thought to consider it, she informed me that she drank no milk. At this time I wasn't very thorough with my questions. She would come and see me about once a month when the symptoms would occur. She would receive two or three treatments, then be on her merry way feeling fine. She would sometimes go for weeks at a time with no symptoms. We finally discovered that she would have ice cream occasionally. When we started paying attention, we found that she would always experience symptoms two days after she had ice cream. Her symptoms are classic, but I also included her case because of the two day onset of symptoms. Most people experience symptoms within a few hours of ingesting foods they are sensitive to, however I have seen several cases that have a two day onset.

Chris, a 21 year old female waitress came in complaining of neck pain after she had been involved in an auto accident where the car she was driving was rear ended. She had never experienced neck problems before. She was in good shape, her x-rays (taken at the hospital) were clean and, as was expected, she responded well and rapidly to treatment. One day, when she came in for treatment, she informed me that her low back was "killing her." She then informed me that her low back had bothered her for years. When it hurt, she would feel pain, burning, and a tearing sensation over her sacrum (tailbone) when she attempted to bend forward from the waist. She had had no accidents or falls before the pain started, except, of course for her recent accident. She had had problems with her low back as long as she could remember. I examined her low back, then began treating her with chiropractic manipulation and physical therapy. She failed to respond. Her case was one of the first ones in which I considered the milk connection. I treated her for two weeks with no response. I was frustrated. Her problem did not make sense to me according to musculoskeletal rules. Her neck problem had cleared up, and at that time, in my limited experience, I had not seen a milk connection case that involved anything but the neck and upper back. I decided to experiment. I took her off milk and her pain went away. She was amazed. I was amazed. After two weeks without milk and without symptoms, I suggested that she return to drinking milk. Her low back pain recurred four hours after she drank her first glass of milk.

She had been trying to get her mother to come see me because she had had a low back problem for years. After her own success with milk, a bell went off in her head. Her mother was a heavy milk drinker. They often had arguments because they couldn't keep milk in the house due to her mother's thirst for it. She took her mother off milk and guess what?

She never became a patient.

Terry, a 32 year old female came in with acute low back pain after falling while water skiing. She consulted me several months before Robert Ester had made me aware of the milk connection. She tested positive for a minor disc injury. After two weeks of chiropractic care, ice, and a low back support, she recovered and was released. One year later she came back in with the same pain, however she experienced no trauma to cause the pain. She said it just got gradually worse until she felt she needed treatment. She also informed me that, although she recovered from her water skiing accident a year prior, her back had continued to bother her. In fact, it bothered her so much that she had quit her job hanging wall paper. Her pain seemed to come and go for no apparent reason. She described her pain as a tearing sensation over her sacrum when she bent forward from the waist (sounds familiar). When she came in one year prior, I concentrated on treating her low back only. Based on what I saw at that time, her x-rays, history, etc., I expected her to recover and be completely symptom free. I was surprised and disappointed that she had continued to have problems. Time alone should have taken care of the problem. I now realized that I was missing something. I asked her if she experienced headaches. She told me she had headaches every day. She figured they were due to stress. She had consulted doctors for years with no results. She had given up on solving her headache problem. I found out that she drank milk nearly every day and loved cheese. I took her off dairy products and treated her low back twice. Her headaches and back pain have completely disappeared.

I ran into her two weeks after she was released. She was extremely happy that her symptoms were gone. She was even happier that she knew why. She had proved the milk connection to herself by trying some cheese at a party. The next day she had a dull headache. In the interim, I had mailed her an article I read on varicose veins. Although she was young and in good shape, she had had varicose veins in her legs for years. She had them stripped once, and assumed she would have to have them stripped again some day. The doctors told her she had inherited the trait from her mother. The article I sent her said that varicose veins can be caused by allergies to foods. Milk was mentioned. I have seen a high incidence of varicose veins in men and women who were allergic to milk. I doubt that her varicosities will get better, because the damage to the valves in the veins is most likely permanent. However, if milk is the cause, they will not get worse, as bad as her mother's, as long as she avoids dairy products.

Gerard, a 27 year old male body builder came to me complaining of left low back pain that radiated to his left groin. He had been suffering with this pain for 5 years. He had been seeing chiropractors for his problem because he found adjustments helped. Although adjustments helped, his pain never went away. He was another patient who came to me as I was just becoming aware of the milk connection. At first he seemed satisfied with the regular chiropractic care I was providing. I was lulled into a sense of satisfaction too, after all, he had been seeing other chiropractors and he didn't seem dissatisfied. However, one day he came in, just before my vacation, and stated his frustration over his condition. And I must admit, I had a hard time convincing him, and myself, that the minor physical abnormalities he had could cause such a persistent problem in an otherwise healthy person. In a moment of desperation, I suggested that he cut dairy products out of his diet. When I returned from vacation he came in to see me. He reported that this was the first time in 5 years he was pain free.

He came in to see me three months later after he had eaten a bowl of ice cream. The pain had returned the following day. Although I treated him for one week, and he reported that he was no longer eating dairy products, his pain decreased, but did not go away. I was puzzled. He was frustrated. Several weeks later, he discovered that he had been eating butter. He usually ate margarine, but his room-mate had purchased butter without his knowledge. When he switched to margarine, his pain finally went away.

Paul, a 63 year old retired police officer came to see me complaining of chronic neck stiffness. X-rays of his neck were a mess. A layman could look at the film and see the severe arthritis. As an officer, he had experienced plenty of trauma to his neck. He reported that his neck was always stiff, and had been for 33 years. He heard cracking and popping when he turned his head. He also reported that his hands would tingle and go numb quite frequently. When he took off his shirt, I noticed a rash of small red spots across his chest at the bottom of his rib cage. He reported that he had had that rash as long as he could remember. He had been seeing chiropractors for 33 years because, of all the doctors he had seen, they gave him the most relief. He was drinking lots of milk for calcium, he told me, and yogurt every day, because "it's good for you and low in calories," he told me. When he cut out dairy products, the stiffness in his neck went away altogether, and his neck no longer popped and cracked, despite the fact that his neck was full of arthritic changes. Three months later, he moved out of the area. The last time I saw him, he still had the rash.

Charlie, a 58 year old man came in complaining of severe neck spasms on the left, mid back pain, and dizziness. He had been experiencing these symptoms for six months. Many times he could not drive to work due to the dizziness. He drank very little milk, but loved cheese and had some every day. When he stopped eating cheese, his symptoms stopped. One month later, he accidently ate cheese on a sandwich. Within 20 minutes he said he felt horrible. He got a headache, his neck ached, and so did his mid back. He also became hyperactive and irritable. His symptoms lasted for four days after the one exposure to cheese.

Dorothy, a 42 year old, overweight woman came in complaining of severe back pain from her neck to her tail bone. She had tingling and pain in both hands and both feet. She reported that both of her hips were "out" and needed to be adjusted. She had headaches every day. She didn't like milk because it "didn't agree with her." She loved cheese.

When she came into the office, she could barely walk. I treated her with physical therapy and instructed her to eliminate cheese and all dairy products from her diet. She returned three days later. All of her symptoms were gone, except some tingling in her toes. Three days after the second visit the tingling in her toes was gone.

Mavis, a 49 year old woman came in to see me complaining of severe headaches, neck pain, left shoulder pain, and pain radiating into both hands. All of these symptoms started 10 years ago when her then husband, now ex, picked her up, not from work, but from the ground, then threw her down. She landed on her left shoulder and was knocked unconscious. She was rushed to the hospital where she was x-rayed and examined. Fortunately, the doctors told her, nothing was wrong. There were no broken bones. She was released. After several months her condition failed to improve, in fact, it got worse. She went back to her doctor. He reviewed her x-rays and, without any other tests, referred her to a neurologist. The neurologist, concentrating on the pain in her hands, diagnosed her problem as carpal tunnel syndrome. Carpal tunnel syndrome is a nerve compression problem that occurs in the wrist, causing symptoms in the affected hand. He suggested surgery, one wrist at a time. The patient decided to have the surgery on the right hand. Following the surgery, the pain in her right hand was worse. The neurosurgeon still wanted to perform the same surgery on the left wrist, and redo the right. The patient refused. A year later, she ended up in the office of an orthopedist. He diagnosed her problem as thoracic outlet syndrome, a nerve compression condition between the neck and upper torso. He wanted to remove a rib and sever a few nerves. Fortunately, she refused.

Finally, this patient decided to live with her pain with the help of daily doses of clinerol. She came into my office for treatment because she had been experiencing more pain than usual, and wanted some temporary relief. She was a heavy milk drinker. In fact, every night she would take her evening dose of clinerol with a glass of milk. This was so she wouldn't wake up with a headache in the morning. However, four or five days a week she woke up with one anyway. She ate ice cream three times a week. She craved cheese. When she gave up dairy products, her symptoms all stopped, despite the drugs and surgery to which she had subjected her body.

Larry, a 27 year old man came in to see me in January of 1990 after he "threw his back out" two days ago, and it just wasn't getting any better. He told me that this happened to him several times a year. He had done a lot of motocross (off road motorcycle racing) riding and had experienced lots of crashes. Even though he had acute episodes only a few times a year, he always felt some discomfort in his low back.

In consulting him about his diet, I discovered that he was what I call a "heavy" dairy user. He loved cheese and ate it daily. He loved milk, consuming a half gallon a day.

I treated him that day and instructed him to avoid milk and dairy products. I also instructed him to avoid sitting, bending from the waist, and lifting, and to apply ice to his low back for 30 minutes at a time, as often as he could. He was to return for treatment the next day. He called and cancelled his appointment.

You see, he had been to chiropractors before. He knew that he usually got relief from having his back "put back in place" by a chiropractor. Evidently, I had either helped him get better, or made him worse. In the latter case, I would be soon receiving a "request for medical records" from another doctor.

Instead, he returned to my office in September of 1990. I was shocked at his appearance. First, it took him about 10 minutes to get out of the truck in which he was a passenger. He walked into the office very slowly, obviously experiencing a lot of pain. This did not shock me, because my secretary had informed me that he was coming in because he had "thrown his back out" again. What shocked me was his weight. He had lost about 30 pounds since I had seen him in January and looked great.

I told him he looked good and first asked him how he had lost the weight.

"All I did" he said, "was eliminate all the dairy products I was eating. That's it. I changed nothing else."

"So, let's get to the business at hand," I said. "What did you do to your back?"

"I was helping my Aunt stack some firewood."

"Pretty heavy stuff, huh?" I asked.

"Not really. It was actually no big deal. I was just tossing small pieces, one at a time, when all of a sudden, wham, severe pain, and I fell to my knees."

"So it really wasn't all that strenuous?"

"No, I was really surprised."

"So you've been totally off milk and dairy products?"

"Ninety-nine percent." (Oooooooh ... that one percent.)

"Have you had any chocolate lately?" (Always my first guess for acute pain.)

"No."

"Any ice cream?"

"Oh, wow! I had some Rocky Road ice cream."

"When?"

"Let's see, you know what? I had some on Monday night."

I always ask for dates and times. His pain began on Tuesday morning at about noon ... rocky road ice cream on Monday night at 11:30 pm. About a 12 hour reaction time. Very average.

Dan, a 35 year old male came into my office with acute low back pain. He had gone to bed the night before feeling fine. He woke up in excruciating pain. He reported to me that he had done nothing physical to justify his pain.

I set the stage, or set him up to consider my point of view:

"So, you didn't do anything like lift a refrigerator, or fall, or something? Doesn't that bother you, or at least make you wonder?"

"Yeah, I guess so. I guess I just have a bad back."

"So, did you eat any chocolate or ice cream last night?"

"Yeah, I guess I did. I had chocolate mousse pie. Why?"

"Do you eat chocolate often?"

"No, just on special occasions."

"Well, I will adjust your back today, because that has worked in the past, right?"

"Yeah, usually one adjustment and I'm okay."

"Well", I said, "I'll be more than happy to adjust your spine. But, I'm going to suggest that you avoid chocolate, at least until you are better."

Pregnant pause.

Incredulous stare.

"Well, I have noticed, over the last five years, that chocolate can cause severe back pain."

"No way."

You know, some days, I just don't want to explain. I told him, "Listen, I'll adjust you, but my additional advice is to avoid chocolate. You don't have to believe me, but that's my advice, okay?"

Well, I adjusted him. I told him to wait two days, then call me if he wasn't better.

He called four months later.

"You know," he said, "your last adjustment really helped. In two days I was fine. Thanks. But you know what? You told me about chocolate, and I really thought you were nuts. But, I didn't have any until last night. And, you know what?"

"No, what?"

"I can't get out of bed. My back hurts like you wouldn't believe. Do you really think chocolate has something to do with it?"

"Yeah," I said. "I've seen it a few times."

June, a 62 year old woman came in to see me in 1986. In 1986 I rarely considered the milk connection. I mainly used it when all else failed. June was experiencing dizziness and her sinuses were bothering her. She had been suffering with the flu for several weeks. Her husband had to help her walk due to her extreme dizziness. He thought that perhaps her dizziness could be alleviated with a cervical adjustment.

It sounded like a good idea to me, so I adjusted her neck. When she sat up after the adjustment, she threw up and was dizzier than ever. She continued to throw up for two days. She had to be hospitalized for dehydration.

Amazingly enough, she came in to see me two years later with the same notion. Again, she was dizzy and thought an adjustment would help. I treated her as a new patient by first taking a symptom survey. She complained of chronic neck stiffness, headaches, cracking and popping in the neck, dizziness, and sinus problems. She reported, upon questioning, that she was drinking two glasses of non-fat milk every day, cheese three to four times a week, chocolate (which she craved) once or twice a week, lots of cottage cheese, and oatmeal with milk three times a week.

Since her problems were chronic, and classic milk connection symptoms, I adjusted her neck and upper back (she didn't throw up), and instructed her to avoid all milk and dairy products and return in seven days. When she returned in one week, she had the following report: She said for years she awoke every morning with stuffed up sinuses. She had to blow her nose for several hours. Her sinuses now were completely clear. After her first visit seven days prior, she experienced fatigue for three days, then her sinuses cleared. Now, she had no dizziness, no neck pain, and no headaches. She said she felt 20 years younger. No more treatment is necessary, except, of course, her own dietary management. I see her now only to say "Hi."

Kristen, a 16 year old female, came into my office complaining of mid back pain, low back pain, and upset stomach. She complained that she was sick and nauseous a lot. She had consulted a medical doctor who ran lots of tests. He found nothing.

She was accompanied on her first visit by her father. In questioning them both about her previous health history, her father reported that she used to suffer with streptococcusstrep infections and tonsilitis. She had experienced shortness of breath on occasion. She and her father both agreed that she was very moody. Her grades were excellent. Her back felt stiff and ached a lot, and she had a habit of "cracking" her back. She was tired a lot.

She reported that she used milk only on cereal, and only once a week. She also reported that she loved cheese and had some every day. She had ice cream once a month, and chocolate only three times a month, she said.

Kristin's symptoms, and the above reporting of her diet, were certainly enough to establish a connection, considering dairy products as the culprit. But I went on. I asked her to describe a typical day in her diet. She was in school, and drank a glass of water in the morning before departing for school. At 11 am she ate lunch at school, usually a grilled cheese sandwich, a cheeseburger, or pizza. She certainly loved her cheese. I asked her what she drank for lunch. She reported that she had chocolate milk every day.

Certainly mood swings can be caused by any food allergen, but the most powerful mood food is chocolate. Although she reported using milk only once a week, and chocolate three times a month, the daily use of chocolate milk made that report inaccurate.

She returned in four days after instructions to avoid all dairy products. She was feeling much better. She was not sick at all, but had some mild back discomfort. She reported on this second visit, that she had been adhering to the diet, except once. She said she experienced stomach cramps five minutes after eating a bag of Cheetos™. She returned for two subsequent visits in the next week. She had successfully managed to avoid all dairy products. She had no back pain and was symptom free. She was released.

No Milk

Mike, a 32 year old male consulted me in 1988 for neck pain and headaches. These symptoms began one day after his car was rear ended. He had never experienced these symptoms prior to the accident. I treated him for two months with chiropractic manipulation and a no dairy diet. He initially had a hard time accepting and following the diet. After all, he had drunk milk his whole life with no problems, until the accident. However, each and every time he suffered a setback during treatment, it was preceded within a few hours by the ingestion of dairy foods. He discontinued treatment.

He returned three years later after he had suffered with acute low back pain for one month. I was surprised to see him and shook his hand. He smiled, and said, "You know, I still can't drink milk without getting a headache. I stayed on your diet for a couple of months after I last saw you, then tried to go back on milk. I got a headache the first time. Every time I have some, I get a headache. So I finally gave up and am living without milk."

He is a weight lifter, and started experiencing low back pain one month after returning to weight training after a year off of training. He was now trying to lose weight. So I asked him if he was using Ultra Slimfast™. (Good guess, huh?)

He was, for about two months now. Chocolate, of course. He reported upon questioning that he drank two or three Ultra Slimfast™ shakes a day, mixed with non-fat milk.

He said, "Yeah, but I don't get headaches when the milk is mixed with the Ultra Slimfast™."

Now I explained to him the phenomenon of changing symptoms. Some patients who initially complain of neck pain and headaches due to milk allergy, will recover after avoiding all casein. After weeks, or months, or years of abstinence, returning to dairy products will cause different symptoms, like low back pain.

Mike returned in two days for treatment. He had stopped the Ultra Slimfast™. His pain was the same and his posture was still antalgic (leaned to the side). I treated him and had him return in two days. His pain was 50% decreased. He was standing straight. He returned in three days, a total of seven days from his initial visit. He was completely recovered, and released.

Pauline, a 72 year old woman, came in to see me complaining of discomfort between her shoulder blades and neck stiffness. She had been to chiropractors for many years for this recurring problem. She wanted an adjustment. That is all the information she gave me.

When I conducted a symptom survey she reported that her hands and feet were always numb. They had been that way for 30 years. She had consulted doctors years ago for this problem, but decided against the recommended carpal tunnel surgery. She reported that her legs felt weak after even the shortest walks.

She never had children because she was unable to. She experienced vaginal bleeding for years, then finally had a hysterectomy. She said she suffered with Brucellosis from age 4 to age 68. She was weak and sick for long periods of time during these years. Her sinuses were always clogged up.

She reported that she drank two to three glasses of milk a day, had cheese three to four times a week, and cottage cheese twice a week. She loved chocolate and ate some three to four times every week.

I adjusted her neck and upper back and instructed her to avoid all milk and dairy products and to return for treatment and follow-up in seven days. She came in seven days later and reported that she had no back pain or neck stiffness. In addition, she reported that her sinuses were clear, and the strength was back in her legs. The numbness in her hands and feet was completely gone. She said she could walk barefooted on her linoleum floor and feel the cracks and the smoothness of the linoleum for the first time.

I always tell patients that they will respond to dietary manipulation in 7 to 30 days. I used to think response time varied with age, older patients being slower to respond. However, it seems more and more that age is not a factor. Pauline is 72 years old. Her symptoms of 30 years were eliminated in less than seven days with successful dietary manipulation.

The following case further illustrates the lack of age as a factor in recovery time.

Chad, a 13 year old boy came in to see me complaining of entire spine pain. His whole back was stiff. (Entire spine pain is a common complaint, and a strong indicator of a dietary problem). He could barely reach his knees when he bent forward from the waist. His knees were always stiff and sore. His mother said she could always hear him walking down the hall, his joints cracking and popping. She said he sounded like an old man. He said he felt like one. He was 5'11" and loved sports. He played soccer, basketball, and pitched in baseball. He would have to lay down for several hours or days after participating in sports. It was customary for him to be carried off the soccer field or basketball court after games.

They had been consulting medical doctors for two years. The doctors said that he was having growing pains and said he would have to give up sports all together. His mother brought x-rays with her that had been taken recently. They were clean and showed no problems.

His mother accompanied him on his visits to the office. She was very concerned. Chad was bent on playing sports and he tried to suffer silently so he could continue to play. She reported that he had ear infections as an infant and was unable to drink cow's milk. He would throw it up. She reported that Chad used to be allergic to milk.

Now, at the age of 13, he drank two or three glasses of milk every day. He loved cheese and ice cream. I adjusted his entire spine and instructed him to avoid all milk and dairy products. I went over the list of foods to avoid with his mother. I instructed her to police his diet. Teenagers are the hardest to control. They both asked if he was to limit his sports activity during the week.

No. Just control the diet.

Chad and his mother returned in seven days. Chad had been good on his diet. I asked several questions about what he had been eating during the week. His and his mother's answers convinced me that he was following instructions. His back was somewhat better, he reported, but not a lot. He had been very active during the week and had suffered with some pain after pitching.

They both returned in seven days. Chad reported that he felt 50% improved. He was able to bend forward farther with less discomfort. His joints still cracked and popped, but not quite as much. Further questioning convinced me that he was successfully avoiding all casein.

He returned for his third visit the following week, 20 days after changing his diet. The cracking and popping in his joints had all but disappeared. He was able to participate in all activities with no pain, although he still experienced some moderate stiffness.

On his fourth and final visit seven days later he reported that he had no pain, no cracking and popping in his joints, and was feeling good. He still demonstrated some decreased range of motion in forward flexion from the waist. I released him with instructions to avoid dairy products for the rest of his life. I repeated those instructions to his mother. I told them both the only draw-back I could foresee for Chad with no dairy foods in his diet would be a decrease in his rapid growth rate.

Patti, a 35 year old mother came in to see me two months after Chad was released. Patti is Chad's mother. She reported that Chad was doing great. He was having no pain. He was a fanatic on his diet. He read all labels and refused to eat at friends' houses when the faire included dairy products. He's an example of how change comes about. New ideas don't become accepted by changing the minds of experienced professionals. New ideas become accepted by teaching them to the new, open minded youth, the students. New ideas become established as the youth spread the word, and as the old, closed minded professionals die out and take their obsolete ideas with them.

No Milk

During Chad's previous sports season, friends and coaches had witnessed his suffering. Patti reported that they often called after watching them carry Chad off the field. They were concerned. This season he has been pitching in baseball, and running off the field. The concerned friends were amazed. "What's the deal?" they asked Patti. Eyebrows became hairlines when she told them his pain was due to milk allergy.

But there he is playing, and how can you argue with that?

Patti complained of neck pain and low back pain. These complaints had been with her for several years and she had just lived with them. But now, she was experiencing what she called a "pulling sensation" on the right side of her throat. She had asked her medical doctor about it, but he wasn't concerned and ignored it. A further symptom survey revealed that she had cracking and popping in her neck, and would get occasional shooting pains over her right eye. She had a hysterectomy at the age of 30 because of a tilted uterus.

She drank milk two or three times a week. She used cheese three or four times a week, especially when Chad wasn't home. She ate salads several times a week with cheese and ranch dressing.

It is so common for a relative to come in with similar problems and a similar diet. So I told her, "Guess what?" I adjusted her spine and instructed her to avoid all dairy products. She returned in three days. On her second visit, she reported that the pulling sensation in her throat was unchanged. Her neck felt better, but her low back was sore. In addition, she now experienced stiffness in her hands and feet and knees. She had never experienced these symptoms before. Backward we were marching into withdrawal.

She returned for her third visit, five days into her new diet. Her low back was better. The joint stiffness was gone. The pulling sensation in her throat remained the same. She was unable to return for treatment due to schedule problems. I called her two months later to ask how she was doing.

"Fine," she responded. (Not a definitive answer for case management.)

I asked how her neck and back and joints were feeling.

"Oh, fine, no problems."

"How about that pulling in your neck?"

"That is still the same."

Not a cure-all.

Florence, a 67 year old woman came into the office on August 26 complaining of severe pain on the right side of her neck behind her right ear. This pain began on August 23 for no apparent reason. She had been to chiropractors before for neck problems, the last time about two years ago. At that time, she reported she "threw her neck out" and saw the chiropractor three times in one week. She recovered and had been okay until two days before coming in to my office.

Florence ate cottage cheese two or three times a week. She used non-fat milk on her cereal every day. On August 22 she consumed chocolate cake and ice cream. I instructed her to avoid all milk and dairy products. I adjusted her neck. She returned on August 28 for treatment. Her condition remained unchanged. She said she could not tolerate the pain. It was excruciating, she reported. I treated her again that day, her second treatment, and checked up on her diet. I was convinced she was following my instructions. She returned again on August 30, four days into her new diet. No change. "I'm going to have to do something about this pain," she said.

"We're doing it," I said. I like to see a response as soon as possible, and we were only four days into Florence's treatment, but she was becoming worried and impatient.

I didn't see her again until September 3, after the Labor Day weekend. Before leaving my office on August 30, I asked her if she had plans for the weekend. A birthday party for a grandchild. Please don't eat any cake or ice cream, I begged. You should be 50% improved or better when I see you on September 3. Wishful thinking.

She returned on September 3 and reported that her condition was 80% improved. She was experiencing some slight neck discomfort. She reported that her condition finally changed on August 31, and had gradually improved. I treated her on September 3 and released her, eight days after changing her diet.

Barbara, a 62 year old woman has seen chiropractors for years. I changed her diet. She got better. She returns every few months complaining of some neck or back pain. Each time we found a dietary connection, each time milk and dairy products. Recently she came in after an absence of six months. She had been consulting a local medical doctor, (one I had referred her to for some of her other problems), because she was getting headaches. He had tried various medications after lots of testing. After several months, he suggested she come see me. Maybe an adjustment might help, he told her.

When she called to make the appointment, she told my secretary to tell me "I have headaches, and it's not milk!!!" She just needed to be adjusted.

When she came in, she told me again, and she was proud, "It's not milk." She gave me the rundown about how her headaches had begun several months ago, and how she had had lots of tests, and tried lots of medications, and she wasn't getting better, and she and the doctor decided she should try an adjustment, so here she was. And it wasn't milk.

Okay. It doesn't have to be milk. It just usually is. Maybe it's something else, but I gotta start at the top and work down. I listened to her diagnosis and her ideas and decided to join the team on this headache problem.

"Let's go over your diet, just to eliminate that possibility," I began. Cautiously. It's not that, you know, but let's be thorough. She thought that would be okay.

After several questions about her use of milk and cheese, etc., to which she proudly denied using, I got down to the standard question: "Are you on any kind of a special diet?"

•

"Well, my husband and I have been on Slim Fast™ for several months, but we mix it with Mocha Mix™."

"What flavor do you use?"

"Chocolate."

Her headaches had begun, to the best of her memory, and as a result of my prodding, shortly after, or around the time that she began her diet. So I told her about chocolate (again) and about the presence of sodium caseinate in Slim Fast™. I was able to convince her to stop using Slim Fast™ and her headaches stopped.

It wasn't milk.

These are sample stories of what I see in my office. Nice stories, huh? Stories like these occur day after day in my office. But there are other stories that aren't so nice. I see patients who don't want to change their diets. Some patients don't want to, but do. Sometimes patients don't respond to treatment. Some patients respond to treatment by following my instructions, then change back to old dietary habits, but don't want to hear about dairy products anymore.

Some patients change their diets and do not respond. Their symptoms remain unchanged. This is not a panacea. There is no such thing. If this was it, I could go live on a farm today.

But my work continues. There's still Barbara and Curt and Kathy. We haven't been able to figure out these cases. These patients, and lots of others, have problems that currently lie beyond my knowledge and experience. So the doubters and the critics can rest assured that this is not a cure-all.

So the 5 - 10% of patients that don't respond to my form of treatment keep me in my office daily. Some of those patients lie to me, some can't remember what they ate, and others have problems that lie beyond the milk connection.

But the truth remains the same. The vast majority of cases of back pain, neck pain, and headaches are due to milk and dairy products. I hereby dedicate the rest of my professional work to those that aren't: to Curt and Kathy and Barbara, and those people I have yet to meet.

Onward into the darkness.

6

Prescription for Health

Most of us have enjoyed the exuberance of youth with seemingly bullet-proof health. As a teenager and young adult, I seemed to have endless energy. I could play hide and seek for hours, running, jumping, giggling all night if my Mom and Dad would let me. I could stay up all night telling stories with cronies, later staying up all night cramming an entire semester into several hours. I could fall off fences, play tackle football for hours. I'd be sore for a few hours or days, then be ready, even eager, for more.

As I got older, the eagerness faded into obligation. Recovery time from injuries got longer and longer. I used to eat like a horse. Couldn't **gain** weight to save my life. Then I turned 30. I didn't play, I worked. I couldn't **lose** weight to save my life.

Health consciousness has grown since my dad was a kid. In the forties, shoe stores had portable x-ray machines you could stand on and see the bones in your feet. Cool. Looking down while all those x-rays poured into your eyes. Not so cool.

We've learned from our mistakes. We've learned that the human body is not bullet proof. Nowadays, most older Americans have given up the careless practices of youth. As we get older, we start to see the price we are now paying for our lackadaisical habits. So, when we turn 30, we realize we need to

213

No Milk

make a conscious effort to get out from behind that desk, off the couch, and into a gym, or at least outdoors to get some exercise. We realize that recreational drugs aren't really that cool, and they go by the wayside, being replaced by jobs and families. When we turn 40 we tire of the chronic cough, the inability to climb stairs without wheezing, so we quit smoking. Several times.

At 50, a life insurance physical has caused a doctor to take off her glasses, tell you about your cholesterol, and order a treadmill test. So now "the wife" is making you drink that watered down milk, you've switched from butter to margarine, only three eggs a week, no bacon, less red meat. You're watching your fat grams. You've got to cut back on your hours at work because you're not handling the stress very well. Gee, you used to love "the heat of battle!"

At 60, after your first heart attack and that long, reflective ambulance ride, you really get serious. You're serious about this now, because the stakes are higher. You want to see your grandkids graduate. You want to keep up with them. You want to stop hurting. You're not ready to die. So you change a few things. You realign priorities. Soon, your friends don't recognize you anymore. You wear jogging outfits. You read labels on the foods you buy. You quit your job that you thought you couldn't live without. You have to buy new clothes because you've finally lost that weight. You're more relaxed. You smile more.

Why did it take so long? Why did we suffer through all the pain? Why did it take until now to straighten out our lives? To get healthy? Because of the exuberance of youth, the resilience of youth, and the exposure to the goodies and the excesses of the American way of life. That's why. Ignorance is bliss. If you never had the goodies, you wouldn't miss them.

As we get older and move through the years, it seems we give up more and more of the goodies as we come to realize the hazards that go with them. When we are young, we are told of the hazards of smoking, but some kids would rather face those risks than the risks of not giving in to peer pressure. The

214

priorities of youth are different. Even though smoking is supposed to be harmful to the lungs, a 16 year old won't feel it. She still has the exuberance of youth. She can run up a flight of stairs with a cigarette in her mouth. No heavy breathing, and looking so cool and grown up. A 16 year old likes to feel the wind in his hair when he pops a wheely on his motorcycle. No need for a helmet. How will the girls know who he is? A helmet is only in the way. Until he bounces his head off a curb.

Young people in this country don't want to give up the goodies. They have so many these days. Our country is so rich. The average family can afford a lot of luxuries. But to afford these luxuries, both parents must work, so the teenagers are home alone managing their own diets and activities. Fast foods, fast cars, and fast sex are pushed at them every day in the media, and seem so desirable. Until they crash, or kill someone, or become teenage parents ... or get AIDS.

A young person loves to give in to the plaid jacketed, smooth talking stereo salesman. Sign here and take that baby home. Take it out of the box. It looks so good on your dresser. Crank it up. Ahhhh, instant gratification. Then those monthly bills start rolling in. The newness has worn off even before the first monthly payment is due. Maybe even a knob or two has fallen off. Gee, only 60 more months of payments. How much did this thing cost, anyway?

Once we've experienced this sort of thing a few times, we learn, we become wiser. We become more willing to hold off on instant gratification until we consider what the long term cost is really going to be.

The same is true in health care, the care of our bodies. Nobody wants to give up something he or she enjoys, and I'm not going to be the one to tell anyone to give anything up. It's just my job to inform, not deny. If doctors could give orders, the Surgeon General wouldn't merely require cigarette manufacturers to put a warning on packages. He would make cigarettes illegal. But this is a free country. At least it's supposed to be. California has managed to pass a helmet law, though, making it mandatory to wear a helmet while riding a motorcycle. Although this will save a few lives, it is an infringement of freedom. A person should do whatever he or she wants with their heads, as long as no one else is hurt by their actions. At the same time, cigarettes and alcohol are legal, but are responsible for hundreds of thousands more deaths. I guess our politicians think liquor is okay. We should be free to drink alcohol by choice. It should be one of our freedoms. We're only hurting ourselves. Right?

Wrong. We all know what alcohol does to people. People fight in bars after drinking. They misbehave on airplanes where the stuff flows freely. Families break up over it. Kids are raised in fear when living with it in their homes. They grow up with problems. It causes liver disease, arthritis, heart disease, and social disorders. Most traffic fatalities in this country involve alcohol. But I guess politicians feel we should be free to use it. I think the laws of the land reflect what our politicians are doing. They're not riding motorcycles without helmets, or smoking marijuana, so they've outlawed those hazardous activities. I guess they'd hate to give up the drinking, the worst poison of them all. Where are our priorities?

It turns out that health care in this country is a matter of giving things up. A cigarette smoker finally realizes that, in order to be healthy, he has to quit smoking. This is difficult to do, and may seem like deprivation. But it's obvious to a non-smoker that the smoker wouldn't feel deprived, he wouldn't have to suffer through withdrawal, he wouldn't have to pay all those dollars to quit, if he simply had not started smoking in the first place. So all you non-smokers should remember that logic when your doctor tells you you need to do without fat, or sweets, or booze, or caffeine...

...or milk.

As we get older and older, the list of things we should give up gets longer and longer. This isn't a conspiracy against older people. The list gets longer and longer for several reasons. First, as we get older and older, so do our bodies. They aren't as resilient as they used to be, and not as resistant to poisons, allergens, and trauma. As symptoms pop up one by one, due to some excess in our life styles, the excesses are peeled off one by one so the symptoms go away. Second, as we get older, we are getting smarter. We are realizing more and more of the things we are doing are harmful. Things that used to seem okay, like standing on an x-ray machine in the shoe store, we now realize are harmful. We now realize that the meat and potato diet is not the best. Cyclamates and saccharine seemed like good ideas at the time. Many medications have been pulled off the market. So we are learning.

The problem, though, is all the red tape. The scientific community needs "proof" before a harmful product can be banned. God forbid we interrupt someone's profit without proof that their product is harmful. We all know that traffic signals are seldom installed because citizens notice a hazard and start writing letters to officials. A few people must die at a poorly marked intersection before a signal is installed. Proof. So until tests prove that a substance is harmful, it stays on the market. With all this scrutiny, you wonder how some of these drugs and additives got past the FDA in the first place.

It goes beyond that, though. Until there is proof, some products not only remain on the shelf, but no warning about suspected problems is even issued. It has taken 60 years for information about MSG to filter into public recognition, and still the scientific evaluation of this poison is "inconclusive." In fact, some products continue to be touted as "healthy," even essential for health, while people continue to experience health problems from the products. "Milk Does a Body Good" is just not true.

So, for Americans to become healthy, they have to give up some things. They need to give up known poisons, like drugs and alcohol and nicotine. They need to give up "suspected" poisons, like caffeine and MSG. They have to give up some things that they believe, or have been told, are healthy. Most people I see don't want to give anything up. They get depressed. "Gee, I already quit smoking. My other doctor says I shouldn't drink, and now this?"

Still others insist on citing examples that go against all we've been taught. Everyone has an aunt or uncle who lived to be 100 smoking a pack a day and drinking a pint of whiskey. George Burns, who's 95, claims to drink 5 martinis and smoke two cigars every day. George Foreman is going strong in the boxing ring at 42, living on cheeseburgers and ice cream. We have no answers for these exceptions. But if you think you can live like these exceptions, what are you doing in a doctor's office?

People come to see me because they are experiencing back pain, neck pain, or headaches, or some sort of musculoskeletal problem. It is my job to help them eliminate these specific problems. At first, they think I'm trying to make them healthy by recommending dietary changes. It is not my job to make them healthy, and I tell them that. I recommend specific dietary changes for their specific problems. To illustrate that point, I often ask if they smoke. If they do, I let them know that they can continue to smoke. I tell them I have not seen back pain or headaches due to cigarette smoking, except in the case of menthol cigarettes. In some people, menthol causes headaches, dizziness, and/or stiffness in the neck. If they don't smoke menthol, I tell them to keep smoking, if they want. It will only kill them, eventually, after they drag an oxygen bottle around for a few years. But it is not causing the problem they are consulting me for.

After a history and dietary analysis, I recommend some changes, usually eliminating dairy products, many times MSG (more and more), and sometimes other foods. Many people look at the list of dairy products and respond, "Wow, you just eliminated my whole diet."

Many patients claim that "everything" has milk in it, or MSG in it. Well, a lot of foods contain milk and MSG, but not "everything." I used to be a big milk drinker, even in the first two years of my practice when I was telling patients to avoid it. I was often asked, "Do you drink milk?"

"Sure," I'd say, "But I don't have any problems with it. I've never had back pain or headaches."

"Well then," they'd respond, "you don't know how hard it is to give it up."

Good point.

So I did. It wasn't hard. It definitely took some concentration, but I was able to do it. I thought, since I had no sensitivity to casein, I would see no changes after eliminating milk products from my diet. However, before quitting, I used to get drowsy in the afternoon, and many times, would take a nap at lunch time. I felt much better after a 30 minute snooze. After quitting milk, that went away. I now write during lunch break. Now, one of the symptom questions I always ask is about a patient's energy level: I ask if they get tired easily.

This is a common complaint among many people, and usually due to food allergy, commonly milk and dairy products. They think it's part of the aging process. "I must be getting old," they say. Well, I think that happens to a minor degree, less than we think, actually (look at Jack LaLane). But not at the age of 32!

Chronic fatigue syndrome has become a popular diagnosis and is a common symptom of food allergy. However, most conventional doctors say it is due to stress, an American way of life, and instruct patients to reduce stress, and get used to feeling tired. It's part of life.

It is my contention, however, that the gradual process of aging does not have to be nearly as drastic as we imagine it has to be. Aging does not have to be a gradual process of deterioration. If it is, poisons and allergens and other problems are present. I treat specific problems by determining, then eliminating specific causes. Many times, I treat a chronic back problem, or headache problem by eliminating milk and dairy products. If the patient doesn't think I'm crazy, they almost always get better, then come back years or months later with a recurrence, or another problem. Sometimes we discover another cause in their diets or lifestyles (although usually it's re-exposure to casein), then add that, or several more substances to their list of things to give up. Many of them have also consulted other doctors for other problems, and have been instructed by them to give up even more foods, or activities.

It seems health care has become a lifetime process of putting out fires as they flair up. Instead, why not practice preventative measures so we don't have the same problems that our friends and relatives have had? Why even start playing Russian roulette when you see the bodies piled in the corner? And if you are playing, why not quit before you join the heap?

Although specific health problems have specific causes, it is my opinion that the treatment for all disease is the same. Hippocrates knew it 2000 years ago when he said:

"The key to health is through natural living."

Antoine Beschamp said it with his five tenants of health: a natural diet, clean water, pure air, a moderate amount of rest, and a moderate amount of exercise.

With more and more people becoming aware and responsible for their health, a plethora of information on the subject is now available. In studying trends in health care, we've learned at least one thing: ideas about what is healthy and what is not change every day. People want to know what to eat, how much to exercise, how much to sleep, what activities are good, which are bad, should they take supplements, and on and on. I have consulted the experts, Hippocrates, Mandell, the McDougalls, Schwartz, the Diamonds, Mendelsohn, John Robbins, my own clinical experience, and my beliefs. I have come up with my own prescription for health, and it is as follows:

1. Eat natural foods.
2. Keep informed
3. Get a moderate amount of rest.
4. Get a moderate amount of exercise.
5. Drink lots of pure water.
6. Breathe clean air.
7. Keep a positive mental attitude.

EAT NATURAL FOODS

"What am I supposed to eat?" This is the most common question I am asked after instructing patients to eliminate foods from their diets. There are plenty of books on diet. Some diets say eat high protein, low carbohydrate, and some say the opposite. Some say to separate the food groups by meals. Some recommend high doses of vitamins and other supplements.

I think almost all the new diet books on the market have good suggestions, and at least some good information. *Eat to Win* by Dr. Robert Haas is okay. The Diamonds' book, *Fit for Life* is good. *The McDougall Plan* by John McDougall and his wife, Mary McDougall, is, in my opinion, the best diet book on the market. *Diet for a New America* by John Robbins explains how we are hurting our health and our environment with the (SAD).. I am not going to give a book report on each one of these diet programs. I have read them all, and more.

I think a lot of these programs make eating seem like a very complex procedure. But I don't think that's how our manufacturer intended it to be. We have become so technical, and so smart over the centuries, that we have made staying alive and eating healthy a technical, complex program with a whole new high-tech vocabulary. I think we're missing the point. We have strayed so far from what Hippocrates said. And we are paying with our health.

The great thing about writing is that I get to express my opinion. The following is based on my ideas, my beliefs, my studies, and my clinical experiences. In other words, it's my own dang opinion.

There are many theories about how we humans got here on earth, and I don't know which one I believe. But the fact is, we are here, and we were designed, by whoever, to live here on earth. Our respiratory systems were designed to take in and use the natural gaseous substances of atmospheric air, our musculoskeletal systems were designed to ambulate around the terrain of the earth. Our nervous systems were designed to sense and react to the air and light and terrain of mother earth.

No Milk

We were designed to drink the natural fluid of the earth, water. And, we were designed to eat what grows on the planet.

A natural diet consists of fruits and vegetables, whole grains, and rice and beans. To drink water and fruit juices. That's it. Any additional verbiage is just an explanation to try to get Americans to give up the rich, fat, unhealthy diet they are used to.

As infants, we were designed to be nourished by our mother's breast milk until our natural instincts told us to stop. Sheep's milk was designed for baby sheep, and cow's milk for baby cows. It is my opinion that we were not designed to suck the fluids out of other animals. It is also my opinion that we were not designed to eat other animals. We have evolved as plant eaters, not meat eaters. Most of our teeth are flat for grinding grains and vegetables. Our hands have developed the opposing thumb, delicate fingers and nails best suited for gathering, not ripping flesh, like the claws and talons of carnivores. Our digestive and salivary enzymes are designed to break down the carbohydrates of plant foods. Our intestines are long, like other herbivores, designed to spend more time breaking down the complex carbohydrates of plants. Carnivores have short intestines for quick digestion of flesh foods.

That's the argument presented by vegetarians, anyway. They're trying to convince people to stop eating animals. The fact is, however, that humans are well suited to eat animals and plants. We are actually omnivores, and to say that humans do not have mechanisms to digest animal foods is just well intended zealousness. But there are still plenty of arguments against eating animals.

At the beginning of this century, the average American consumed 216 pounds of grain and 182 pounds of potatoes per year. Beef, poultry, and dairy products were "treats" that were consumed only on rare occasions. By 1985 the grain and potato consumption of each American had been cut in half, while the consumption of beef is up 50% per person, and the consumption of poultry is up a whopping 280%!

With the development of mechanized farm equipment, transportation, and refrigeration, farming became a process of mass production, as was the production of animal foods. Now 90% of the grain produced in our country is used to feed livestock, and only 10% is for human consumption. To produce one hamburger requires 16 pounds of grain. The grain used for the hamburger, if eaten instead, would provide 21 times more food energy and 8 times more protein.

It takes 2500 gallons of water to produce one pound of meat. It takes 4000 gallons of water to produce one day of food for a meat eater but only 300 gallons of water to produce a day of food for a vegetarian. In fact, most of the water in this country is used to irrigate crops to feed livestock for meat eaters to consume. Producing food for animals to be eaten does not make sense, and it is causing the poor health conditions in our otherwise rich country. Chopping down the forests so cattle can graze is upsetting our ecosystem.

We have already discussed how misleading labels are on packaged food. Have you ever seen a label on a package of meat? How do you know what that animal ate before he was slaughtered? What medication was he on? Was the meat injected with steroids or growth hormone? What are you putting into your body when you eat that meat?

Do you need more to convince yourselves to stop eating animals? Well, since this book is my opinion, I have to express it. The logic I have just gone through ought to be enough, but my thinking goes beyond logic because I have animals, and I love them.

What is it that makes some people want to go out and kill "game?"

I have a friend who claims to be a liberal thinker, a conservationist. He has a garden, he rides a bike, he opposes the killing of whales, and he loves to hunt. That doesn't make sense to me. Sorry.

Why do some animals deserve to be hunted and killed? I guess those are the lucky ones. At least they have a chance.

No Milk

Most animals that are killed for food are raised in captivity, then herded up to some Neanderthal with a gun or a hammer, to be slaughtered so we can eat them.

But what is hunting all about, anyway?

The thought is that some animals will over-run us and upset the ecology, the balance of nature. They're in the way of condos and freeways and crops used to feed us and other domesticated animals that we plan to eat. We must control their populations by chasing them around the woods, a gun in one hand, a beer in the other, shooting them, taking a picture of them under our boots, then taking them home and mounting their carcasses on our walls. This is sport, I guess.

Did God (or whoever you can relate to) create a world that demanded that we use our superior intelligence to go out and kill innocent animals? Is it because the animals can't protest, they can't verbalize their pain? Are we so unfeeling that we can't look into their eyes and see what they feel?

Not me.

I have three dogs and two cats. If you have animals that you love, you know what I'm talking about.

Look into their eyes sometime.

To me, animals are our examples, our redeemers.

They do not speak.

They do not judge.

They only love.

They have souls.

They are God's creatures and we can learn from them.

I do. Every day.

I chose dogs and cats because that's who I live with. To me, they represent the animal kingdom. They are no better than squirrels, or deer, or pigs, or cows. They're all the same. All these creatures have souls.

Look into their eyes. Can't you see it? Look into a cow's eyes. Have you ever seen a more docile, peace-loving creature than a cow? Do they deserve to die at our hands because they cannot speak to protest?

No.

Those who eat flesh are being punished with poor health.

So a healthy diet does not include meat or dairy products. Many patients complain that reading labels is a pain. I have given them a list of foods to avoid. Manufacturers use misleading labelling ploys, so we don't even know what is really in the food we are buying. Many of my patients complain that it takes four hours to go grocery shopping anymore. Many of them ask, "Isn't there a short cut, or a general guideline that makes label reading easier?"

Yes there is: **If it has a label, don't buy it.**

There, that's pretty simple isn't it.

Too limiting?

Okay. If the label has more than four ingredients, don't buy it, and if any of those ingredients are chemicals, don't buy it. Avoid packaged foods. If it comes in a box or a can, don't buy it. If it has a label, it means the law has required the manufacturer to admit what they are putting in your food. I don't want any doubt about what I'm eating. There's enough doubt already due to poor labelling requirements. Babies like to find out what things are by sticking them in their mouths. Hopefully, as adults, we're smarter than this. Eliminate all doubt. If you don't know what it is, don't eat it.

What does that leave?

Like I said before, rice, beans, vegetables, fruits, whole grains, water and fruit juices. Use whole grain rice. White rice has been stripped of the husk, where all the fiber is. Organic produce is best. Home grown is even better. Most produce in the stores today has been chemically treated with pesticides, fertilizers, and other chemicals used to make them look more attractive. Most large cities have stores that sell organic produce. If you live in a small town that offers no organic produce, wash all your produce thoroughly with soap and water. Most of the chemicals used are oil based and will not come off when washed with plain water.

Subscribe to *Vegetarian Times* and *Organic Gardening,* magazines that know a lot more than I do. Read *Prevention* magazine, and *The McDougall Plan* where you'll find healthy recipes. These books will explain in further detail why you should eat a healthy diet.

Many patients ask me about supplements. I have a standard reply when a patient asks me if he or she should take vitamins or supplements. I ask: "Are you taking vitamins now?"

If they say "yes" I ask them if they feel better for taking them. If they do, I tell them they should continue. If they don't feel any better, or feel worse, I suggest that they save their money.

Most supplements are natural substances that the body uses for daily functions. Many vitamins are water soluble. If you take too much of a water soluble vitamin, your body will dump the excess in the urine. Some vitamins will cause a reaction when overused, like niacin, vitamin B3. Many people have experienced the intense flushing of the face, and itching that accompanies their first dose of niacin as a supplement.

Other vitamins are fat soluble, and can accumulate in excess in the fatty tissue of the body, or in the liver. Vitamin A, for example, is a fat soluble vitamin found in fish. The recommended daily allowance for vitamin A is 10,000 units. When Shackleton and his men where exploring the polar ice cap, they hunted and ate polar bears. Polar bears live on fish, and store about 8 million units of vitamin A per ounce in their livers. When Shackleton's men feasted on polar bear liver for dinner, they suffered. Their skin fell off and they died. They overdosed on vitamin A.

There are other problems with vitamins. A common vitamin C tablet contains 500 mg of vitamin C. 500 mg of vitamin C is not visible to the human eye, but it must exist in tablet form so we can see it, handle it, and put it in our mouths. So my question is, what is all the rest of the stuff that makes up the tablet?

Sometimes vitamin companies use "inert" fillers to bulk up the tablet. Sometimes these inert fillers aren't so inert to some people.

There are plenty of supplements on the market. Most of them are carefully formulated, then carefully produced, and carefully marketed with one goal in mind: to make money. A natural diet requires no supplements. So some people think, since they eat on the run, they need supplements. They don't have the energy they need to make it through the day without caffeine and vitamins and fast food. So I guess vitamins and supplements are designed for the new age person on the go. If you live on cheeseburgers, you should take vitamins.

That is the typical medical mentality: "Eat whatever you want and just take your medication." Do what you gotta do and take vitamins. I recently read in a *Woman's World* magazine a column called "Ask the Doctor." A woman asked the doctor why she got panic attacks after eating Chinese food. He mentioned MSG then went on to say "Panic attacks can be treated with tranquilizers and psychotherapy. Mild MSG allergies can be controlled with antihistamines while severe cases can be life-threatening if adrenalin is not administered."

How about avoiding MSG? He didn't mention that.

So if you live on cheeseburgers, should you take vitamins?

No. Stop eating cheeseburgers and get on a natural diet.

✦ KEEP INFORMED

One of the first things to do before you go to the doctor is to investigate your condition. Many times, in the act of seeking information, the answer to your problem can be found before you have to pay a professional.

You must be informed about your condition before you speak with a doctor, otherwise, he or she can tell you anything. Without some knowledge, the doctor can lie to you, suggest treatment or advice that is obsolete, or doesn't work. There is no way you can ask intelligent, pointed questions to help manage your case unless you are informed. In *Confessions of a*

Medical Heretic, Dr. Mendelsohn says you should know more about your problem than the doctor, before you see him. Many people believe that doctors know everything. We don't.

As a doctor, I feel the most important thing I can offer my patients is my experience. I'm not smarter than my patients, I just have more experience in my area of training, and therefor, more information. I have seen certain symptoms, problems, and pain complexes, over and over again. All doctors do this. If they are paying attention, they can recognize trends. After practicing for enough years on enough patients, doctors can begin to realize what works and what doesn't work for each particular problem, despite what the textbooks say. Textbooks are just guidelines. They point the doctor in the right direction (most of the time). They are not the law. They get old. They change. Based on a doctor's experience, he can tell you what he's seen with patients who've had similar problems.

No doctor can predict 100% of the time how a patient will respond to treatment. But after a doctor has seen similar cases enough times, she can, based on that experience, more accurately predict how the patient will likely respond and what he or she can expect in the future. A doctor doesn't have to predict, he can just be honest and open with the patients and tell them about his own experience with their particular problem: what he has seen, what works, what doesn't work, how long recovery usually takes, what will aggravate the problem, etc. I usually describe similar cases to my patients in story form. Patients can usually relate to that and get a sense of security about their condition and their future. This sense of security has a definite effect on their recovery.

Any treatment program must be a team effort by the doctor and the patient. Each player must do his or her part. Face it, if the team fails, only the patient loses. The doctor always gets paid. In order for the patient to do his or her part, she must become informed about her condition. I know everyone is not informed about medical matters, but even so, becoming educated does not require extensive formal education, or reading through complex medical textbooks.

To become informed, first, talk about your condition with friends, relatives, and associates. Talk with people who have had the same problem. When you do, pick their brains. Find out the history of their condition, what caused it, what helps, what doesn't help, what aggravates the problem, what recovery was like, how long did it take, what the doctors said and did. This information is invaluable. Some doctors will tell you it's not, because it's not a professional opinion. All the better. No money is involved, so you'll probably get more straight forward and less confusing information. Remember, no doctor knows more about a human body than the owner. Ask some owner who have been through your experience. It helps a lot. Ask anyone in AA (Alcoholics Anonymous).

Second, I think everyone should subscribe to at least one health magazine. I think the best is *Prevention Magazine*. This is a monthly periodical, about the size of a *Readers Digest*. Each issue is chocked full of helpful information about health with a holistic approach. Read it from cover to cover. Keep informed before you have problems. It will keep you out of doctors' offices. You don't want to go there. There are sick people there. Besides, most times the doctor is just going to give you some poison. This isn't health care. It's modern medicine, and it doesn't get people better.

Let's Live is another monthly health magazine that is very helpful. There are lots of other weekly and monthly periodicals on medical self help. I think they are all good. They are like doctors' opinions — more is better. Remember, the doctor's main purpose is to inform you. In managing your own case, you want mainly to gather as much information as you can. You don't have to believe everything you read. You don't have to try all the remedies you read about. You don't have to do what the doctor tells you to do. That's right. The days of "doctor's orders" are over. Your body is not in the military. It belongs to you and only you. Don't let a doctor intimidate you by refusing to treat you unless you follow his or her orders. If that is his attitude, he obviously doesn't know his job. If a doctor gives you orders, dump him, and find a caring doctor who wants to help you, not control you. Before you submit your precious body to any form of treatment, gather lots of information and opinions, then **you** decide what to do about it.

Your home library should contain several books to help you keep up on, and manage your family's health. Every home should have a medical dictionary. A medical dictionary is necessary so you can understand what the doctor is talking about. There are many on the market. I like *Taber's Medical Dictionary*. It is small and complete. You don't have to spend a lot of money. If you want to be real frugal, check out the used book section at college book stores, or yard sales and swap meets.

Another item sometimes found at garage sales is another book called *The Physician's Desk Reference,* the PDR. This book is the drug bible. It lists all the prescription drugs on the market, their indications, contraindications, side effects, chemical structures, dosages, etc. It even has pictures of the pills. The PDR picks up where the doctor left off with, "Here, take these." This book comes out each year in a desperate attempt to keep up with the pharmaceutical companies. You should own a relatively new one, especially if you insist on taking drugs.

I also recommend owning a *Merck's Manual*. This is a reference book that lists diseases and conditions, their signs and symptoms, and treatment. This book will keep you from going to the doctor needlessly. For example, shingles is a viral disorder that causes a nerve irritation and a rash. It usually occurs on the torso, on one side following along one or more ribs, and is very painful. If you go to the doctor, she will probably order x-rays and blood tests, then prescribe a special, expensive, topical lotion, or calamine lotion. You'll be better in two to three weeks. If you stay home and do nothing, you'll be better in two to three weeks.

Finally, I think all families should own an *Anatomy Coloring Book*. Sounds pretty elementary, but it is, in fact, an excellent anatomy book of the entire human body. Each organ system is presented separately with pictures to be colored. All the parts are labelled. Each system is accompanied by a brief, understandable description of the structure and function of the parts, and the system as a whole. If your doctor tells you you have a problem with your pancreas, you can quickly look it up, find out what it is, what it looks like, where it is, what it does, all in terms you can understand.

There are no cure-alls in modern medicine. When penicillin was first introduced, it appeared to be a cure-all. Before penicillin, people with infectious diseases like pneumonia, had to suffer with their symptoms until their own body healed itself, or they died. Penicillin and other antibiotics became such apparent cure-alls that they have become over used and misused. Most antibiotics are antibacterials, that is, they kill bacteria. Many people feel obligated to go to the doctor when they have a cold, or the flu. These disorders are usually caused by viruses. Antibiotics have no effect on viruses. The only way to kill a virus is with a vaccination, and there are very few viruses for which a vaccination has been developed: small pox and polio are two. Flu shots are a joke. There are so many different strains of the flu virus, new ones develop every year, that there is no way a flu shot is going to be specific for every different strain. When you get a flu shot, you most likely will get the flu. People are funny, though. My Grandmother is a strong believer in doctors and medicine. She has a lot of each. She gets a flu shot every year, and every year she gets the flu. Last year she blamed it on not getting the shot soon enough.

Antibiotics are powerful drugs that, when used correctly, work wonders. But remember, every drug has side effects. Antibiotics are either injected or taken orally. One way or the other, they end up in the bloodstream. They don't seek out the infectious bacteria that is causing your symptoms, if indeed that's your problem. They kill all bacteria they contact. You may have heard the term, "broad spectrum antibiotics." These are not real specific. They kill all kinds of bacteria. There are plenty of good bacteria that live in our bodies and serve useful functions. Many bacteria keep yeasts (like candida albicans) in check. They also control other populations of bacteria and viruses. Antibiotics do not spare these good and necessary bacteria. When broad spectrum antibiotics are used, the delicate balance of the body's internal flora and environment is upset. The population of Candida can go unchecked and out of control, causing gas in the intestines, vaginal infections, skin rashes, etc. Many doctors know this and prescribe antifungals with antibiotics, especially with women who are susceptible to yeast infections. Broad spectrum antibiotics are like Agent Orange in Vietnam. Agent Orange was not specific for the enemy, just ask some Vietnam Vets.

Amoxicillin is a broad spectrum antibiotic. The PDR says, "... the possibility of superinfections with mycotic (fungal) or bacterial pathogens should be kept in mind during therapy. If superinfections occur (usually involving Enterobacter, Pseudomonas, or Candida), the drugs should be discontinued ..." New antibiotics are being developed every year. Why? Because overuse of antibiotics has caused superinfections and the adaptive development of superbacteria, and super viruses.

If you feel obligated to go to the doctor, or take your child to the doctor, for a cold or the flu, he or she will most likely feel obligated to write a prescription. That's what they do, you know. My advice is, if your symptoms are tolerable, let your own natural healing mechanisms take care of the problem. Do what your body tells you to do. If you feel tired, sleep. If you are thirsty, drink water. Take care of yourself. Don't pour poison into your body, it only confuses matters. Those confusing matters are why a PDR is so thick. The largest section in the PDR on most drugs is the "Adverse Reactions." That alone should tell you something.

When you go to the doctor and she decides you need a prescription, ask her if the drug is active against the infectious agent she thinks you have. You would be surprised how many times doctors prescribe antibiotics for viral infections. The drugs are completely useless in that situation. Ask her what side effects you may experience. Ask her what the contraindications are.

After you have bugged the doctor with questions, bug the pharmacist. Pharmacists are usually much more willing to spend time telling you what they know about the drugs they dispense. Then, before you put it in your mouth, go home and read what your PDR has to say about the drug you are about to take. When you weigh the symptoms of your complaint in one hand, and the side effects of the drug in the other, you can make a much better, more informed decision about what to do.

Any time a doctor recommends surgery, get a second opinion. Surgery is a radical invasion of your precious body. Surgery is a last resort. For musculoskeletal problems, start out with a chiropractor (after you have informed yourself about your problem). Chiropractic care is conservative care. Chiropractic has been a controversial issue throughout its existence, much less today, however, than it used to be. Chiropractors are like everyone else — there are good ones and there are bad ones. The important point is, chiropractic is well founded, well proven, powerful, and conservative. Before considering a doctor, consider the tools he or she uses. A chiropractor uses his hands, a surgeon uses a knife. Which one would you use first? Common sense tells you to consider the more conservative alternative first, then work towards the more aggressive approach. Besides, a chiropractor will refer a patient to a medical doctor if that is indicated. An M.D. will almost never refer to a chiropractor. And they'll brag about that!

Chiropractic first, drugs second, surgery last.

Before you leave a doctor's office, or his care, for any problem, you should know three things:

1) What caused your problem?

2) What can be done about it?

3) How can you prevent it in the future?

The most common medical experience provides only the second answer:

"Here, take these."

By far, the best way to treat any medical problem is to avoid it. First, become educated about your body and learn how to keep it healthy. Most people go to a lot of trouble to read owner's manuals on new, expensive equipment or toys they buy. They place a lot of value on their new possessions and treat them right. Many times, though, these same people get a little slack with these possessions a few years down the road when the new wears off. The same is true of many people and how they treat their bodies. When they were new, mama took great care to give them the best food, bed, clothing, and education available. You didn't take over total control until the old bod was 18 years old, had a few dents, ran a little rough at times, etc. Your priorities changed. There seems to be no time to exercise or eat right or get enough sleep when you have to work 40 or 50 or 80 hours a week.

The human body and its health and well being is a finely tuned mechanism. In order for it to run trouble free for an entire lifetime requires more than mere occupancy. Maintenance and prevention are the keys to a successful relationship with your body and health. Keeping abreast of new developments and thoughts by keeping informed is necessary.

REST

If there were a manual for the human body, it would say that the mechanism must be rested for a certain period of time in each 24 hour period, depending on use. How much rest is necessary?

There are two kinds of rest: sleep, and rest. Sleep is rest with loss of consciousness. Rest is rest while conscious. Sleep is for the nervous system, or software to recuperate. Rest is for the body, or hardware to recuperate.

There are plenty of books and articles and opinions on the theory of sleep, how much is necessary, what position is best, what kind of sleeping surface is best, etc. The most important variable of sleep is time. Sleep is a cyclic phenomenon that is dictated by the central nervous system. Secretions of substances in the brain occur at approximately 90 minute intervals that raise and lower brain activity. This occurs constantly as long as the brain is alive.

It has been determined by physiologists that the effects of sleep occur mainly for the benefit of the nervous system. The other body systems do not require "sleep" per se, as the nervous system does. They do, however, require rest, which will be discussed shortly. The nervous system will usually tell you when sleep is required. A feeling of fatigue will set in. People will notice that they suddenly have an inability to concentrate. Children, as most parents know, are pretty obvious about needing sleep. When small children stay up too late, their behavior changes. Some kids become suddenly hyperactive, or giggly, they act silly, they spurt out sentences or songs that don't seem to make any sense. I call it "short circuiting." Their activity is not unlike that of a pocket calculator when the batteries run low. All kinds of nonsensical numbers flash on the display when the batteries are "tired."

When the nervous system is weary, you may have had the experience of mixed and combined thoughts about the experiences of your day, or recent memory, that come together in nonsensical patterns. "I signed a contract today with our cat at my son's school." So sleep is required for the nervous system to rest. This will explain why a day of no physical activity, but intense concentration (like the SAT tests) will make you very sleepy, or a day of intense physical activity will be followed by the inability to fall asleep. If the brain is not fatigued, you will have trouble getting it to shut down and let you sleep.

The 90 minute cycles of brain activity are what dictates the amount of sleep required. When sleeping, brain activity oscillates between shallow sleep (or paradoxical sleep, also called REM sleep, rapid eye movement), and deep sleep, then back to shallow sleep — all in approximately 90 minute cycles. The ideal time to awaken is in the shallowest sleep, right after dreaming. Most of us have had the experience of waking up right after or during a vivid dream. A person is most rested when gently aroused out of shallow sleep. Conversely, a person awakened from a deep sleep will feel groggy, and, most likely, tired for the rest of the day, even after many hours of sleep.

The best way to be awakened is with a very mild stimulus that will allow the body and brain to awaken out of shallow

235

sleep, but leave a person in deep sleep alone. Some stimulus of light or sound should be used.

A loud or obnoxious alarm clock will go off at a predetermined time and awaken you whether you are in deep or shallow sleep. If a clock radio is set for low volume with mild music, it will let you sleep if you are in deep sleep, but arouse you peacefully when you come into shallow sleep. I prefer to leave the blinds open at night, so I'm awakened by the morning light as the sun comes up. If the blinds are shut at night, I won't awaken in time, due to lack of stimulus. If you must arise before the sun, use a clock radio, or put a mild light on a timer. Einstein learned to function very well on about four hours of sleep, or about two complete cycles. The object is to get in at least two complete cycles and awaken gradually while in shallow sleep to a mild stimulus, either light or sound. Following these rules will give your brain the best quality rest.

What kind of sleeping surface, or bed is best to give the physical plant, the hardware, it's needed rest? I am asked quite often which is better, a regular bed, or a water bed? In my opinion, there are no hard, fast rules about beds. I have one rule, or guideline: If you usually wake up in the morning feeling great, rested, and with no stiffness or soreness, don't change beds. If you wake up feeling stiff, or sore, or lousy, change beds. Don't rush out and spend $1000 on a new bed before you know ahead of time that it's what you need. A 15 minute nap in a bed store is not a sufficient test. So sleep around. If you wake up stiff and sore no matter what kind of bed you sleep on, the problem probably isn't the bed. If you're having problems sleeping, experiment and pay attention to your diet, environment, etc. One of the classic symptoms of milk allergy is morning muscle stiffness. Do you sleep well on vacation, but not at home? If so, the problem could be any number of things, like stress, allergies to plants or animals you have at home, feather pillows, polyester sheets, flannel sheets, air fresheners, etc.

The following case is an example of an investigation into a sleeping problem. A 27 year old male complained that he woke up every morning with a stiff neck and a headache. Dietary manipulation didn't help. (See, it's not a cure-all). We tried changing pillows, eliminating down feathers. There was no change. We tried changing his sleeping positions. No change. He stopped treatment for one week while he went on a skiing trip. When he returned, I asked him how he slept, and how he felt when he woke up while on vacation. He reported that he had no headaches or neck stiffness while on vacation, but after just one night at home, his symptoms returned. To me, that pointed to a problem in his house, or his hometown. Further questioning revealed that his headaches began this winter. I asked him if he ran his furnace at night. He did. I had him sleep one night with the furnace off. He woke up feeling fine, no headache, no stiff neck. I felt we were getting close. His own investigation revealed that the air intake for his furnace was in the garage where he had stored several gallons of solvent. When he took the solvent out of the garage, his problem disappeared.

The point of this story is, if you are having sleeping problems, investigate and experiment with the bed, the pillow, the air, the diet, etc. Keep experimenting until you wake up feeling fine. A relentless search may take some time, but will usually uncover the problem.

The best positions for sleeping are on the back and/or the sides. There are plenty of experts who will argue about which side is best, right or left. But side sleeping is most stressful on the shoulders. If you want to cause right shoulder problems, always sleep on your right side. Otherwise, try to divide your sleeping time between right and left sides and your back. To ease pressure on your back, place a pillow between your knees when sleeping on your side. The least stressful position for the spine is a semi-fetal position, with flexion of the knees and the hips. This can be best accomplished on the sides, although with pillows under the knees, this position can be attained on your back. Looking at the body from the front, the spine should be in line. That is, don't let the head tilt up towards one shoulder, or down towards the other while side sleeping. The correct pillow thickness will get the job done. When sleeping on your back, use only a thin pillow behind the head or under the curve of the neck. Don't use two or three pillows so your head is flexed so far forward that your chin touches your chest.

Avoid stomach sleeping. When sleeping on your stomach, you must turn your face to the right or the left in order to breath. Most people always turn the same direction. This creates limitation of motion in the opposite direction, and stress on the joints in the neck. Stomach sleeping also puts pressure on the low back by increasing the sway in the low back. This is especially true on waterbeds and soft mattresses where the body and pelvis sink deeper.

If you find yourself sleeping in positions that cause you problems, start to change your sleeping habits. However, don't be impatient with yourself. Changing lifetime habits takes time. Start by spending some time at the beginning of each night, when you first get in bed, in one of the low-stress positions. When you feel you must move out of this position into a problem position that you are used to, go ahead. Then in the morning, before you get up, place yourself again in a low-stress position. As time goes by, try to gradually increase the time at night and in the morning spent in good positions. If you have a hard time breaking yourself of the habit of stomach sleeping, place a pillow under your stomach. This will flatten the sway in your low back and reduce some of the stress until you can learn to avoid that position altogether.

Fortunately, your body, like your nervous system, will tell you when it needs a break. Get in tune with your body. Listen to what it tells you. When you are full, stop eating. Don't clean your plate just because that's what you were taught. Next time, take smaller portions of food. The digestive system needs rest too, and it will tell you when it does. When your muscles ache or tire, stop using them. If your joints start to ache or stiffen, stop using them. Let them rest.

Sleep and rest are essential for good health, and despite what you may have heard, are not that complex. Listen to your body and try to give it what it is asking for. It will last longer and run better.

EXERCISE

Exercise means different things to different people. In a nutshell, movement is essential for good health. The cardiovascular system depends on movement for blood to return to the heart from the arms and legs. All the joints of the body must go through a full range of motion each and every day. If you don't use it, you lose it. A full range of motion is what you create and use for yourself.

World class women gymnasts have a greater range of motion in their joints than most people, because they have stretched the joints beyond normal range of motion so they can perform the graceful moves they use in competition. At the other end of the spectrum is the 70 year old retiree who spends most of his or her time sitting, watching TV, always looking straight ahead. You've probably seen them changing lanes on the freeway, using the "hit or miss" technique, staring straight ahead, instead of turning their heads. Through underuse, they have created a limited range of motion. When sedentary people become weekend warriors on the touch football field, or basketball court, they force their joints to move beyond the range of motion of their normal activities. They hobble to work on Monday, or go to the chiropractor.

When a healthy person breaks an ankle and has it casted for six weeks, guess how much that ankle moves when the cast comes off? Not at all. Zero. Studies have shown that when a joint is immobilized, adhesions and scar tissue begin to form within four hours. Certain musculoskeletal injuries require immobilization in order to heal. Broken bones must be immobilized until the new bone growth of healing can tolerate stress. Torn muscles must rest until sufficient healing has taken place to avoid reinjury. Very few other musculoskeletal injuries, though, respond to bed rest and immobilization. Many doctors love to prescribe bed rest for injuries they don't know how else to handle. I have seen patients who were ordered to bed for six weeks because of back pain.

No Milk

I see two classic cases that are typically mismanaged by immobilization. Acute low back pain is most often caused by an injury to the disc, the pad between the vertebra. The usual medical treatment, after lots of x-rays, CT scans, etc., is a prescription for anti-inflammatory medication, muscle relaxers, and six weeks of bed rest. Most of the time, the pain will subside after six weeks ... until the patient tries to get up, or after he or she has taken a few steps, or bent over one time. Then, the pain is back. Six weeks down the tubes. If a low back case is not a surgical one (herniated disc), I recommend chiropractic care, which is **mobilization** possibly a low back support, ice, **walking**, and, of course, dietary manipulation. Generally, patients find that the first few steps of walking are painful after periods of immobility, like sitting in a car, or sleeping. But after a few steps, the pain usually subsides.

Another condition that is usually mismanaged by immobilization, is frozen shoulder, or adhesive capsulitis. This shoulder condition is usually caused by a direct blow to the shoulder, or a quick jerk (come on, honey), or overuse. Many times, there seems to be no apparent cause, and guess what? The shoulder joint is often affected in cases of casein sensitivity. A patient with this condition is unable to raise his or her arm without pain or difficulty. They find it difficult to take off and put on blouses and shirts. They have trouble brushing their hair. It hurts to sleep on the affected shoulder. I can always tell when they have been to an M.D. first. They walk into the office with x-rays in one hand, and the other arm in a sling. The immobility provided by the sling has caused the shoulder to become stiffer and more painful. I prescribe exercises that move and stretch the shoulder joint, exercises that break up the scar tissue in the joint, exercises that hurt! Even though these exercises hurt, mobility is usually increased within hours and days, even in long term cases. The pain is slower to leave, but as mobility increases, the pain decreases and is eventually gone. When the shoulder is immobilized with a sling, scar tissue continues to form, and the condition becomes worse. The medical solution for this doctor induced immobility is surgery.

¶ Regular mobility and exercise is essential for good health. This doesn't mean you have to join a health club, become a runner, sign up for aerobics three times a week, or start lifting weights. If you are young and aggressive, participate in aggressive sports. Take aerobics, lift weights, play racquetball, run marathons. The most important thing is to choose an activity that you enjoy. If exercise is rote and boring, you will eventually quit unless you are masochistic. Exercise is essential for mobility of the joints and for strengthening the cardiovascular system. In my opinion, the very best exercise is walking. After all, that's what we are designed to do. A good brisk walk of one hour, every day, will mobilize the joints, exercise the heart, exercise the lungs, clear the brain, and get you from point A to point B without overstressing the joints. Swimming and bicycling do the same thing.

Exercise, in some form, must be done every day. For a healthy cardiovascular system, the heart rate must be pumped up to about 80% of maximum. There are lots of high tech gadgets that will allow you to calculate and count your heart rate, blood pressure, steps per minute, walking speed, distance, etc. etc., ad nauseam. Keep all that junk at home so you can enjoy the walk. Your walk should cause you to breath hard and work up a sweat. It doesn't have to be any more complex than that. A couple of brisk, 30 minute walks a day will accomplish that. I think everyone should walk more, anyway. Once you get in shape, you'll find it's not so bad to walk on some of your shorter errands. Even your long ones.

Exercise is not only good for the body, but is good for the mind and the soul. Exercise is a great outlet for tension and stress. Because of this, I do not recommend stationary bikes, tread mills, or rowing machines unless absolutely necessary. And if exercising indoors is necessary, I would recommend changing things, realigning priorities, or moving. Get outside, breath the fresh air, look at and appreciate the beauty of nature. You're alive and free in the greatest country in the world, the USA!! Yahoo!

If you don't think that will make you feel better, try it!

PURE CLEAN AIR

Air is essential for life. Without it, there is no health, because there is no life. Air is a mixture of oxygen and nitrogen. Air also contains water vapor that assists the lungs in absorbing oxygen. As oxygen is taken in through the airway and lungs, toxins and carbonic acid are expelled. This gaseous exchange is necessary for life and health. When people ingest substances their bodies can't use, like preservatives, processed foods, tar and nicotine, etc., the expulsion of carbonic acid is hampered. Carbonic acid concentration in the blood increases, causing acidic blood and susceptibility to inflammation and infection. That's one reason why smokers are sick more often than non-smokers with colds, coughs, infections, etc.

Pure, clean air exists in only one place — outside. If you work inside, you are breathing in air that contains all the rejected carbonic acid, carbon dioxide, toxins, and germs of everyone in the building. The air has been "conditioned" for your comfort by being sent through heaters and air conditioners, through tubes and filters. It's conditioned all right, it's artificial, unnatural. If you really want to breath some foul air, stay in a hospital sometime. If you don't get sick, feel lucky.

Everyone should get outside every day to breath fresh air. I know, in lots of places it's not that fresh. If you live in an area with dirty air, like the L.A. basin, move. If you live in the desert, grow lots of plants around your house and in your house. Plants produce oxygen, essential for healthy tissues and active brains.

PURE CLEAN WATER

I mentioned before that there are no cure-alls known in modern medicine. There is no pill that will cure arthritis or heart disease, and no elixirs or potions that will prevent aging. However, the best potion known to man to aid in health is water. It is present on our earth in abundance right now. The human body is composed mainly of water. The blood and brain are 4/5 water. Water is necessary to transport nutrients and waste materials through the blood and digestive tract. Water keeps all the mucous membranes moist and functional. Water provides a medium for the elimination of waste through the lungs, the kidneys, the skin, and the bowels.

Disease does not grow in pure, healthy blood. Moving pure water in and out of the body is essential for pure blood. Did you ever notice how some people are sick a lot, and others are not? When flu epidemics strike, not everyone gets sick, not even everyone who is exposed to the germ. Disease will grow in impure blood, but not in pure, healthy blood.

Okay, we all need water, but how much? People who eat lots of meat and animal products, sweets, salt, and processed foods don't get much water from these foods. In addition, they are ingesting lots of toxins that must be eliminated. With little or no water in the diet, these toxins hang around in higher concentrations in the blood and digestive tract, interfering with nutrient exchange and elimination. They are also absorbed into the tissues causing organ dysfunction, unhealthy skin, unhealthy odors, fatigue, and generally, an unhealthy condition that leads to disease. People who eat lots of fruits and vegetables, which are high in water content, don't need as much additional water.

As a general guideline, people should drink one ounce of pure water per pound of body weight each day. So, a 200 pound man should drink 200 ounces of water per day to help maintain healthy tissue, digestion, elimination, pure blood, and optimum health. Another advantage of lots of water in the diet, is that it occupies space and therefor helps satisfy hunger. The hunger sensation is set off by two mechanisms: the amount of sugar in the blood, and the fullness of the stomach. When you keep the stomach full by drinking lots of water, you are not as hungry for as much food. I suggest taking a large, 32 ounce plastic cup to work, for those who work. Keep it on your desk and sip on it all day long. Empty it two or three or four times a day.

Drink purified, bottled water. Tap water has been treated with chlorine and fluorine. While tap water is okay to bathe in, the chemicals in it are not natural substances and should not be ingested. These impurities, and others found in tap water, interfere with normal absorption and elimination and have been implicated as possible causes of disease. It has been suggested that chlorine may be a major cause or factor in interfering with calcium absorption, therefor contributing to osteoporosis.

Water has many applications when your health has become compromised. When you are sick, drinking lots of water increases elimination of the poisons in your body that are making you sick. When the immune system is fighting infection, it produces toxic waste and damaged tissue that must be eliminated. Water is excellent for transmitting heat or cold to the body. The application of heat to the skin increases blood flow to the area of application. Conversely, the application of cold, or ice, decreases blood flow to the area of application. Hot water will warm the body faster than anything when you are cold. Ice will lower body temperature faster than any medication.

I am asked quite often what is best for musculoskeletal injuries, heat or ice? Most people insist on using heat when they are injured because it feels good. Textbooks say to use ice for the first 24-72 hours after an injury, then use heat. That recipe doesn't always work. When the body is traumatized to the point where tissue is damaged, blood vessels in the area are also damaged. Blood vessels are everywhere. When muscle tissue is torn from overuse, or ligaments are torn, the small capillaries that supply blood to them, are also torn. Many times, swelling will be evident in the area of injury due to blood leaking into the tissue from damaged capillaries. It usually takes 24-72 hours for the body to repair these torn vessels. So the theory is, apply ice to slow circulation to the injured area while these vessels are being repaired. This will reduce the amount of blood that is spilling into the tissue, and decrease swelling. Ice is also analgesic, that is, it will reduce the pain caused by the damage with its numbing effect. Once the blood vessels have healed, apply heat to increase blood flow. With the increased blood flow, nutrients are brought in for repair work, and the toxins and waste products are hauled away to be eliminated.

My suggestion is this: when in doubt, use ice. Ice will never make your condition worse, unless of course, you have frost bite, or circulatory problems, like diabetes. Ice is a very powerful tool. It decreases inflammation and swelling, and it numbs pain. If your pain is sharp, use ice. If your back pain hurts when you cough or sneeze, use ice. Heat is good for relaxing sore muscles, or for loosening muscles prior to stretching. Other than that, heat has very little therapeutic value. It is mainly palliative, that is, it feels good. Heat will not usually have a great overall effect on the healing process other than to feel good.

POSITIVE MENTAL ATTITUDE

There are plenty of things in this world over which we have no control. Taxes, jobs, kids, and relationships can make you feel pretty helpless at times. But there is one thing in this world over which you, and only you, have total, absolute control. And that is, your state of mind. No matter what is going on around you, you always, always, always, always have a choice of whether to be happy or unhappy. In my opinion, the main purpose in life is to be happy. All the other things are just vehicles to get us to happiness. This is such a great country because the U.S. Constitution says one of our inalienable rights, not privileges, but **rights** is "the pursuit of happiness."

But there seems to be a lot of unhappiness around. A lot of folks seem uptight. Nations go to war. Unhappiness always seems to come about because somebody took offense to something that somebody else said, or did. But, as Ken Keyes says in *Prescription for Happiness:*

"You don't have to respond to Anything by taking offense."

Offensive acts or statements don't have to be acted upon in a negative way. In fact, they don't have to be acted upon at all. If a person is so unhappy that they have to act offensively, let it be their problem. Don't share in their unhappiness. Just do like Bobby Ferrin says, "Don't worry, be happy."

Worrying is a non-productive, negative emotion. Choose not to worry, because, after all, worrying won't change anything. If your boss tells you on Friday that he wants to see you "on the carpet" first thing on Monday morning, you can choose to worry about it, if you want. You can ruin your whole weekend if you want. But that won't change what will happen on Monday. So don't worry. Be happy while you can. Most times you ruin your whole weekend imagining the worst, then find out it's nothing. Maybe the boss wants to give you a raise, or a promotion.

A positive mental attitude helps everything. Did you ever notice that when you're happy and confident, everything seems to go your way? That's no accident. You, and only you, have the power to create your own destiny. It has been widely published that a positive mental attitude helps in the healing process. I've had patients come into my office thinking, based on what they had heard, that I was a great doctor and they just knew I could help them. Believe me, with that kind of attitude, their problem is half solved.

Most people know lots of stories about people who had terrible accidents and were severely injured. Doctors told them they'd never walk again, or run, or play the piano, but of course they did, and went on much further to heroic accomplishments.

The body is controlled by the mind. Make it do good things.

Despite all the technological advances in health care and modern medicine, the very best way to be healthy is to avoid as many of these technological advances as you can. The human body is not a perfect system, but nigh-on-to-it. Despite man's attempts, I feel the system cannot be improved. The key to health is to maintain the system as it was designed. Eat the natural foods that grow on the planet. Don't eat the animals and don't drink their milk. Exercise, rest, drink lots of pure water, breath clean air, and get outside every day and enjoy this wonderful life. We don't need supplements or electronic monitoring devices. Stay in tune with your body. Don't analyze it and weigh it and measure it so much. Don't step on scales. You'll know when you lose or gain weight by how you look, how you feel, what people say, how your clothes and jewelry fit.

I think the health care professions are just beginning to learn about the significance of diet and its relationship to health. If you are having health problems that the doctors can't seem to figure out, experiment with your diet. Cut out the bad foods and the foods you are eating every day, and see what happens. You will see that you are indeed what you eat. When you learn some of your own connections, share them with your doctor so he/she can learn and share it with others.

Who knows? Maybe you'll be someone's Robert Ester.

7

Last Word

So there it is: Casein is the main cause of neck pain, back pain, and headaches. And this is the truth.

You know, I think the reason we are here on earth is to seek and discover the truth. And it jogs the mind when you get a glimpse of the truth. I mean the real truth.

I believe in God, and I hope that I get a glimpse of Him, or Her, before I die. Oh, I've seen the wonderment of God, and all the beauty of Nature, and, even though I have a scientific mind, I am not so arrogant to think that all around me couldn't have come from a Creator greater than Man. I have been taught to pray to God for thanks, and in time of need. But I don't go to church. I've been there a lot, and I didn't see God there. But I have two sisters who have met God, and we all know people who make that claim vehemently.

They're fanatics. My sisters are pretty mellow now, after years of trying to convince me of the truth they have seen. I guess there comes a point when you don't always share the truth, because minds are closed to it, and you tire of the rebuff. I know people who could benefit from what I know, from the truth I have seen, but they don't call or come around anymore, because they're tired of hearing about it. Some of them are relatives, and I have to bite my tongue when they tell me about all the tests their doctors are performing, all the medications they're taking, and the diagnoses they have received. This medical charade is not approaching the truth. No where near.

I bet my sisters bite their tongues a lot when I'm around, and see how I live, not approaching the truth that they have seen. I can identify with my sisters now. I used to think they were fanatics. Now I'm one. Because I was so fortunate to have gotten a glimpse of the truth. A fanatic is one who has seen the truth, and is trying to share it with others who have not seen it, and deny that it is true.

All of the recent studies on food allergy, those by Mandell, and Foreman, and Randolph, all mention the closed mindedness of the medical community. It seems baffling to us that such a simple and useful notion meets with such resistance. I mean, closed minded doctors, and patients, for that matter, don't just scoff. They get angry! Many patients who have heard my story, later consult a "real" doctor and ask him about it: "Can milk cause back pain?"

"Absolutely not!" is the usual reply from these all-knowing doctors.

I would ask these professionals, "How would you know? Because you haven't heard it before? Because you haven't read it in your medical journals? Have you ever looked? Have you tried manipulating diets and looked for results?"

Basically, they've never looked, because if they had, they would have seen it. Because it is the truth. It's like trying to argue with someone about your name.

"My name's Dan."

"No it's not!"

This book is another explanation of bio-ecology. Dr. Theron Randolph saw that foods caused disease in 1943. Most doctors have discounted his work. But others, the minority by far, checked it out. They saw it too, and now there is accessible information on the subject.

However, I searched diligently for these studies, for the work of others who had seen what I was seeing, and had trouble finding anything. I read a lot, but most people don't. My neighbor was talked into taking the L.A. Times. He had to cancel the paper just so he could get in his driveway! Like most people, he doesn't have time to read.

This information is out there if you look hard enough. Many studies have been performed by lots of professionals, and all the results point to the same thing: **Most disease is dietary in origin, and most people don't believe it.**

It's okay to not believe that most disease is dietary in origin. It's okay to not believe that most back pain and headaches are caused by milk and dairy products. But at least check it out, for God's sake. What do you have to lose? This is not a recommendation to undergo a risky medical procedure, or to spend a lot of money. The worst that can happen is nothing. All cases of back pain and headaches should start with a dietary analysis, and usually the elimination of dairy products. Most cases will be solved with this approach. Not **all** cases, but the vast majority. At least start here before you scoff, or get cut, or drugged. Most cases of back pain and headaches that seek conventional medicine get poor results.

This book has been about the relationship between musculoskeletal pain and foods, mainly milk and dairy products. My work has just begun, but already I have seen so much that needs to be shared, that I felt obligated to write this book, and tell you what I know so far. I wrote everything that I knew on the subject down once in 1988. The information was shaky. My glimpse of the truth, at that time, was just that, a glimpse. My description of what I had seen in 1988 was erroneous, on many counts, because I didn't have enough information. My writing was bad, not that it's much better now. The truth in 1988 was but a glimpse, but now, I have managed to corner it and get a better look at it. My 1988 treatise, and this one, are descriptions of a phenomenon that is the truth.

But as sure as I am that this is the truth, I am also sure that the facts will change as additional information is gathered. I am just beginning to realize that I think I have stumbled upon a monster. That monster is cow's milk being consumed by

humans. I have seen thousands of cases of back pain and headaches due to cow's milk. I have seen many other musculoskeletal problems caused by cow's milk. I have seen cancer develop
in people who were allergic to cow's milk. I have seen heart
attacks, varicose veins, inflamed breasts, hearing problems,
seeing problems, and on and on. I have seen virtually every
system become involved as cow's milk courses through the
human body and does it's damage.

It wouldn't be so bad if cow's milk wasn't pushed as health
food. We actually fell for that. But the truth is, cow's milk is
probably the unhealthiest food on the planet. For people, that is.
I think the discovery that cow's milk is the number one cause
of disease may not be far off, depending on how powerful the
dairy farmers are, and how much resistance they offer.

Perhaps we will find that animal proteins, and disease and
viruses spread from animals to humans, are the causes of most
serious disease processes, and that probably the single most
powerful aid to health will be to stop eating animals and animal
products, like their milk.

It's frightening to think of what the future will uncover. As
more and more doctors and other professionals wander out onto
the fringe of medicine, we will see more and more of the truth.
I have seen but a glimpse. I have some pretty heavy questions
wandering around in my head:

Does leukemia occur in people who don't drink cow's
milk?

What percentage of heart attacks are immediately preceded
by the ingestion of MSG?

Maybe there will eventually be a cure for allergy. I have a
friend who's a chiropractor. He is learning how to cure allergy
with Applied Kinesiology. Using this technique, electrical
changes are affected so weaknesses are eliminated. The theory
is that, after successful treatment, the patient can be exposed to
previously reactive allergens with no reaction. Treatment
begins with the question, "What are you allergic to?"

No Milk

To me, the most difficult part of allergy work is determining the answer to that question. If the patient knows that, the solution is already evident. If you're allergic to milk, don't drink it! Now maybe this new technique will cure allergy, I just don't know, and quite frankly, I just don't care. Maybe allergy shouldn't exist in a perfect body. I may come to that sort of work down the road. I'll watch for it. I'm young and I will persist at this work as long as I live. I have much to learn.

We need more eyes and minds searching for the truth. Right now, most conventional doctors are working hard, searching for answers. A lot of experts are looking for the needle in the haystack. But guess what? The needle isn't in the haystack. Look over here, guys.

I will sit down and talk with anyone, anytime, about the fact that milk and dairy products cause most back pain, neck pain, and headaches. I am as sure of that as I am of my name.

I've read that the saying of the nineties is going to be, "I could be wrong."

About the causal relationship between casein and back pain and headaches, I prefer to steal a line from the Eagles' tune, "Victim of Love."

"I could be wrong ... but I'm not."

Sources

1. Colbin, Annemarie, *Food and Healing*, Ballantine Books, N.Y. 1986

2. Foreman, Robert, *How to Control Your Allergies*, Larchmont Books, Atlanta, Georgia, 1984

3. Hunter, Beatrice Trum, *Gluten Intolerance*, Keats Publishing, New Canaan, Connecticut, 1987

4. Mandell, Marshall, *Dr. Mandell's 5-Day Allergy Relief System*, Pocket Books, N.Y. 1979

5. McDougall, John A. and Mary A., *The McDougall Plan*, New Win Publishing, Clinton, N.J. 1983

6. Oski, Frank, *Don't Drink Your Milk*, Mollica Press, Syracuse, N.Y. 1983

7. Schwartz, George R., *In Bad Taste, The MSG Syndrome*, Signet, a division of Penguin Books, N.Y., 1988

8. Winter, Ruth, *Poisons in Your Food,* Crown Publishers Inc, N.Y. 1991

9. Keyes, Ken, *Prescription for Happiness*, Love Line Books, OR 1986

10. Robbins, John, *Diet For A New America*, Stillpoint Publishing, Walpole, NH, 1987

11. Robbins, John "Animal Agriculture and the Water Crisis" *The Animals' Voice* , Volume 4, Number 2, April/May 1991

12. Klaper M.D., Michael, "The Real High Cost of Meat," *The Animals' Voice,* Volume 4, Number 2, April/May 1991

13. Mendelsohn M.D., Robert S., *Confessions of a Medical Heretic,* Warner Books, N.Y., N.Y. 1979

14. Haas, Robert, *Eat to Win*, Signet Printing, 1985

15. Diamond, Harvey and Marilyn, *Fit for Life*, Warner Books, N.Y. 1985

16. Selye, Hans, M.D., *The Stress of Life,* McGraw Hill, New York, 1956

17. Challem, Joseph and Lewin, Renate, "Emerging from a Schizophrenic Haze," *Let's Live,* November 1988

Index

255

Index

For additional copies of

No Milk

please enclose a check or money order for $12.00 for each copy.
This includes all taxes and handling charges.
Be sure to also include
your **name** and **return address,** printed clearly.

Mail your order to:
Wilhelmina Books
Svl Box 8354
Victorville, CA 92392

We would also appreciate any anecdotes or questions about
your case. Please mail to the same address.